FOUR WOMEN AGAINST CANCER

Also by Alan Cantwell , M.D.

THE CANCER MICROBE

QUEER BLOOD

AIDS AND THE DOCTORS OF DEATH

AIDS: THE MYSTERY AND THE SOLUTION

FOUR WOMEN AGAINST CANCER

Bacteria, Cancer and the Origin of Life

Alan Cantwell, M.D.

Foreword by John Steinbacher

Aries Rising Press
Los Angeles

Copyright © 2005 by Alan Cantwell
First Printing June 2005

Aries Rising Press
P.O. Box 29532
Los Angeles, CA 90029

ISBN 0-917211-33-2

Library of Congress Control Number 2005904012

Cover and interior production by Casa Graphics, Inc.

Printed in the United States of America

Printed on acid-free paper

10 9 8 7 6 5 4 3 2 1

In memory of four
extraordinary women
scientists who uncovered
the germ cause of cancer—

Virginia Livingston,
Eleanor Alexander-Jackson,
Irene Corey Diller,
Florence Seibert.

"When science cannot be questioned, it is not science anymore: it is religion."

—Tony Brown
(Tony Brown's Journal)

TABLE OF CONTENTS

Acknowledgments

Some of the ideas and research contained in this book go back to the early 1960s, and it saddens me that so many people who were instrumental in guiding me along the way are now gone. Foremost are the four preeminent women cancer microbe workers you will meet in this book, and my mentors J. Walter Wilson, M.D. and Lyon Rowe, M.D., and the late Eugenia Craggs.

A special thanks to my microbiologist friends. To Dan Kelso for his expertise in growing bacteria and his encouragement over four decades; and Lida Mattman, Ph.D., for her brilliant research in the field of cell-wall-deficient bacteria.

I also owe a great debt to Kaiser Permanente and Southern California Permanente Medical Group, especially the Pathology Department, who supported my studies during the 29 years I worked in the Department of Dermatology in Hollywood.

I thank Lawrence Broxmeyer, M.D., for prodding me to write this book about Virginia Livingston. Over the past decade of my retirement, David Jones (editor of *New Dawn* magazine) and Joan D'Arc and Al Hidell (editors at *Paranoia*) have been exceedingly kind in welcoming my controversial medical writings in their publications. Similarly, Trevor Marshall, editor of the on-line *Journal of Independent Medical Research*, has been tremendously helpful in allowing me to present additional cancer microbe research on the Internet.

Without the encouragement of The Cancer Federation and John Steinbacher, I would never have attempted this book. Thank you, John.

A special thank you goes to Carlanne Hall for her faith in me, and to Ed Garren who is always there for hugs and computer malfunctions, and to George Cabrera for his spirit.

As I recently learned firsthand, there are few things more life-altering than a cancer diagnosis, especially when it affects family. Last year, my partner of 31 years, Frank A. Sinatra, was diagnosed with prostate cancer. As fate would have it, this gave me my first opportunity to successfully hunt for bacteria in this cancer. His prognosis is excellent, but this unsettling experience has made me even more determined to bring the knowledge of the cancer microbe to a wider audience.

And lastly I wish to thank you, dear reader, for your willingness to read a book about a "cancer germ" that the medical community claims does not exist. I leave it to you to decide for yourself.

Alan Cantwell
Hollywood, California
February 9, 2005

Foreword
Virginia Livingston, As I Knew Her

As the founder of the Cancer Federation in Banning, California, I am delighted to write this foreword as a commemoration of the centennial of the birth of our dear friend and supporter, Virginia Livingston, M.D.

The Cancer Federation was founded in 1977. Its goal was to set new agendas to influence medical science and to provide community support for cancer patients. From the beginning we were not interested in the status quo.

In our view, the present state of cancer research is neither humane nor holistic, and our aim is to be life affirming and sustaining. Our challenge was to create new opportunities for cancer research, particularly in the field of cancer immunology.

Over the past 28 years we have realized that we cannot succeed alone. Thus, we have allied ourselves with a network of like-minded progressive people and organizations. This provides both diversity and accountability. In addition, we have sponsored classes, radio and television programs, conferences, media education, outreach programs, grief counseling, and other services to provide community support for cancer patients and their families.

There is no one that exemplifies the pioneering spirit and dedication to cancer research and immunology more than the late Virginia Livingston.

Born on December 28, 1906 in the small coal-mining Pennsylvania town of Meadville, she was the daughter of family physician Herman Wuerthele. At the beginning of the century it was unheard of for a girl to aspire to be a medical doctor, but Virginia was no ordinary woman. As a physician and scientific researcher, her revolutionary ideas about cancer would cause her enemies to regard her as one of the most notorious female doctors of the twentieth century—and make her admirers hail her as one of the greatest scientists of all time.

After high school she attended Vassar College, a premier institution of higher learning for women, where she graduated with honors. Following in her father's footsteps, she received her medical degree from New York University in 1936. Never the shrinking violet type, Virginia was an outspoken and spunky young woman. For example, at a dinner meeting where she was introduced to Dr. Jack Goldberg, Commissioner of Hospitals for New York City, she bitterly complained about the fact that there had never been a female chief resident in any of the city hospitals and thought it was definitely time for a change.

Within ten days she was summoned to Goldberg's office and informed that she was being offered the job of chief resident in charge of hospitalized prostitutes with venereal disease. Years later in her 1972 book, *Cancer: A New Breakthrough*, she admits she was somewhat taken aback because this was not exactly the position she had in mind. But nevertheless, she decided on the spur of the moment to accept the post, assuming it had to lead to something better.

As fate would have it, the position nurtured Virginia's great compassion. Instead of finding the work unpleasant, she became quite attached to the diseased and socially discarded women under her care. During this tenure she also had the unusual opportunity to treat some patients with tuberculosis and leprosy. Both diseases are caused by infectious "acid-fast" bacteria. Remarkably, her experiences with these diseases would later greatly assist her in uncovering the secrets of similar acid-fast bacteria that she discovered in cancer.

A decade later, as a school physician in Newark, New Jersey, she encountered a case of scleroderma in a school nurse. Scleroderma is considered to be a disease of unknown cause characterized by diffuse hardening of the skin, and often accompanied by ulcerations of the skin due to constriction of the blood vessels. The nurse's ulcerations reminded Virginia of certain ulcerations seen in leprosy. Out of curiosity, Virginia took some skin tissue scrapings from the nurse's nasal ulcerations, put them on a slide and colored the tissue with an acid-fast stain, and slipped the slide into her microscope. To her amazement there in the stained tissue were acid-fast bacteria similar to what she had been trained to observe in TB and leprosy (now more commonly known as Hansen's disease).

Virginia called the unusual bacteria she discovered in scleroderma, Sclerobacillus Wuerthele-Caspe. Later, similar acid-fast bacteria in scleroderma were reported at the Pasteur Institute in Brussels, and also by Alan Cantwell, a Cancer Federation Life Member and dermatologist who worked at Kaiser-Permanente in Los Angeles. I have had a keen interest in scleroderma for many years. My own father died of this awful disease in 1950.

In laboratory experiments the scleroderma bacteria were injected into chickens to determine the effect. Amazingly, Virginia and her colleagues were sometimes able to induce cancer tumors in some of the chickens. This eventually led to Virginia's discovery of similar acid-fast bacteria in a variety of different cancers, as well as in certain other inflammatory and degenerative diseases.

Two distinguished women researchers who were to have a great impact on her life were Cornell University microbiologist Eleanor Alexander-Jackson, Ph.D. and Irene Diller, Ph.D., a cell cytologist and animal experimenter at the Institute for Cancer Research in Philadelphia and also editor of the biological journal *Growth*. Associating with Virginia would sometimes cause trouble in their professional careers, especially for Jackson.

Jackson's boss at the Cornell lab was Dr. Wilson Smilie, an intransigent old curmudgeon, who gave Eleanor strict orders to keep that nutty Jersey woman out of his institution. With the door to Cornell blocked, Virginia, stubborn and determined as ever, simply hunkered down in her lab in her basement at home in Newark, where she continued her long and lonely investigation into the microbial cause of cancer. It was safer for Diller and Jackson to collaborate from a distance.

During the war years Virginia was married for a second time to Dr. Joseph Caspe, a noted chemist and fourteen years her senior. A first marriage to a talented but alcoholic journalist broke up before she finished medical school. In 1943, the Caspes became proud parents of an adopted baby girl named Julie. However, there were health and financial problems in the family. Joseph Caspe struggled with severe financial reversals and had a near fatal coronary. As a result, Virginia was forced to take several jobs to make ends meet.

With time her husband's health improved and so did their finances. They were able to rent a large house in Newark with the first floor used as an office where she could see patients, with the basement converted into a laboratory.

In her scleroderma research she was using products manufactured by Abbott Laboratories. The pharmaceutical company offered her a research grant, but stipulated she would have to be affiliated with a college. She was offered a post at Rutgers University as head of the new Rutgers-Presbyterian Hospital Laboratory for the Study of Proliferative Diseases. She also managed to get a series of grants from the Damon Runyan Fund and even the American Cancer Society. In later years, the Cancer Society would condemn her as a quack doctor. With her fine facilities at Rutgers and the esteem that came with it, Virginia was soon elevated to Associate Professor in the

Rutgers Bureau of Biological Research.

Working on her own, Eleanor was able to obtain cancer tumors for bacteriologic study from Memorial Hospital, which was part of Cornell University. She confirmed that the microorganisms were present in all tumors. In culture the microbes were intermittently acid-fast and highly variable in size and shape (pleomorphic). They were similar to the unusual growth forms that Eleanor had previously seen in her extensive research with the bacteria that cause tuberculosis and leprosy.

Virginia, Eleanor and Irene were able to fulfill "Koch's postulates," the series of essential experimental steps that are required to prove that a specific microbe produces a specific disease. With proof that the microbe was not a contaminant, Virginia and Eleanor were able to classify the "cancer-causing agent" as belonging to the order *Actinomycetales*.

By mid-century Virginia had surrounded herself with colleagues who declared that there was indeed an infectious bacteriologic agent that was associated with cancer. Their paper written by Virginia, and a pathologist, a microbiologist, a microscopist and an electron microscopist is the landmark paper that introduced the cancer microbe to the medical world. Titled, "Cultural properties and pathogenicity of certain microorganisms obtained from various proliferative and neoplastic diseases," it was published in the December 1950 issue of the *American Journal of the Medical Sciences.*

The discovery opened the floodgates of abuse from the cancer establishment that would plague her for the rest of her life, just as it had plagued many cancer microbe researchers of the past.

One of Virginia's most implacable enemies at that time was the powerful Dr. Cornelius Rhoads, head of Sloan-Kettering Memorial Hospital, one of the leading cancer treatment hospitals in the country to this day. Rhoads' work was concentrated on finding chemotherapeutic agents that would destroy cancer, and he was so cocksure of the rightness of his views that he would brook absolutely no interference or questions from anyone. On more than one occasion he arrogantly declared: "When the cause and cure of cancer is found, I will find it." He died without finding either one.

The first media attack on the cancer microbe research came following a triumphant conference in Rome in 1953 where Virginia presented her research before some of the world's most prominent biologists and physicians at the Sixth International Conference of Microbiology. Returning by ship to New York, she was confronted at the dock by newsmen bombarding her with questions. The next day reports in the *Washington Post* and the *New York Times* appeared, featuring cancer doctors violently opposed to her findings of a so-called cancer germ. A spokesman for the New York Academy of Medicine was quoted as saying: "This is an old story and it has not stood up under investigation. Microorganisms found in malignant tumors have been found to be secondary invaders and not the primary cause of the malignancy."

From that point forward, there were lost grants, accusations and intimidations surrounding the cancer research; as well as continuing ups and downs in Caspe's chemical business ventures. Everything seemed to go downhill on the East Coast, as chronicled in her 1972 book. Finally, Joseph Caspe was offered a job with a firm in Mexico, and Virginia decided to pull up stakes and relocate near San Diego, where her father had retired and where her only sister lived.

By 1954 Virginia was living in Los Angeles with her daughter. With all avenues of research closed to her, she again found work as a school physician, treating such patients as the young actress Natalie Wood. One day at work Virginia developed neck pain, which by evening had turned into excruciating agony. Her arms and legs began to ache, and she decided it must be polio. Fortunately, she was found to not have a serious form of the disease and recovered in two weeks. This was just a few years before the Salk and Sabin polio vaccines became widely available. The following year Virginia relocated to San Diego.

In 1955 the Salk vaccine produced by Cutter Labs in the San Francisco bay area was released to the public. I was living in the Bay area at the time, and I clearly remember the scandal that erupted when ten deaths and 191 cases of paralytic polio were caused by the actual vaccine. I was an insurance adjuster for the company that insured Cutter, and I played a small role in that event.

Remarkably, Virginia with the aid of her sister, Dr. Lillian Ravin, and her father, were the first physicians in San Diego to administer polio vaccine to school children. The only casualty was Virginia's daughter Julie, who became desperately ill from the vaccine and nearly died.

Meanwhile, her husband's business venture in Mexico had ended on a sour note and he arrived back in San Diego with no funds. He wanted to relocate back to the East Coast, but Virginia refused to go with him. Instead, she financed his trip back and took a new job with the San Diego Health Association.

Joseph Caspe wrote frequently, but obtained a position with the government of Haiti that necessitated spending much time there. One day Virginia was notified that her husband had been found in a New York hotel room, dead as a result of a diabetic coma. Virginia was back to square one.

Fifty years old with a daughter to support, she had not practiced general medicine for many years. Pulling herself up by the bootstraps, she went to work at a clinic that was one of the first to operate on an insurance plan.

This was very controversial at the time and doctors who joined such an association were not allowed to join the medical association. Being an older woman in a male-dominated clinic, she claims she was forced to work like a dog, seeing patients on an assembly line with ten minutes allotted to each patient and fifty scheduled patients a day.

Despite the heavy workload, it was a great opportunity to learn about cancer. In those days before chemotherapy, there was little recommended treatment except surgery, which seldom helped, and even diagnosing cancer in its early stages was difficult.

At the clinic Virginia met her third husband, Afton Munk Livingston, M.D., or A.M. as he liked to be called. Head of the Eye, Ear, Nose and Throat Department, and a competent and gentle Mormon, Virginia fell madly in love and eventually married him and converted to his religion.

Even though she was a workhorse, Virginia's health was never robust and, in 1962, she suffered a severe heart attack. Rushed to a cardiologist, her pulse could not be detected. For over a year she was a total invalid, unable to walk unaided. Refusing the usual treatments for her condition, including surgery, she instead went on a strict regimen of massive doses of vitamins and a diet very low in sugar and fat.

Eleanor suggested a vaccine for Virginia, based on the work of English physician W. M. Crofton who claimed the vaccine was helpful against the buildup of cancer bacteria. There was no way to prove it, but Virginia always believed Crofton's vaccine saved her life, and she continued to take it occasionally for the rest of her life.

Never one to be idle, she utilized her convalescence to mull over her earlier cancer papers and animal experiments. She noted that a number of the animals had developed "interstitial collagen disease" following injections with bacteria derived from cancer. They also developed lesions in their hearts. Even baby mice who were injected showed heart muscle damage. This led to an autopsy study of people who died of heart and blood vessel disease, and the identification of previously unrecognized acid-fast bacteria in heart disease. In 1965, this research report, co-written with Eleanor, was published as "Mycobacterial forms in myocardial vascular disease" in the *Journal of the American Women's Association.*

That same year Livingston, Jackson and Diller all took part in the Science Writer's Seminar conducted by the American Cancer Society in Phoenix, Arizona. Virginia had no idea what kind of response she would get from the press, but the ensuing local newspaper stories were kind in their coverage. Unfortunately for Eleanor, someone from the Cancer Society reportedly contacted Columbia University, where she was now employed. Shortly thereafter, she was terminated. From now on, anyone who inquired about Dr. Livingston's work was told by the American Cancer Society that her work was controversial and "unproven." Even though Virginia was never officially questioned by anyone at the Society about her medical activities, she was slandered for the rest of her life. It was hard to believe that she once actually had a grant from the ACS in the early years of her cancer microbe research. Now the Society claimed Livingston's cancer microbe did not exist.

I first encountered Virginia Livingston when I was assigned to do a story by the *Anaheim Daily Bulletin*, where I was employed as a reporter and education editor. At the time I knew little about cancer. Earlier I had worked with the famous news columnist Walter Winchell in connection with the Robert Kennedy assassination, and I had written a couple of his stories under his byline. Winchell was the founder of the Damon Runyan Cancer Fund, and told me about the difficulties of running an independent cancer organization. I quickly learned through him that the American Cancer Society has a policy of attacking cancer groups, as well as physicians and researchers, whose cancer claims they do not like.

I arrived in San Diego and met Virginia and her husband A.M. in an older house in the city that served as their clinic. This was the beginning of what was to become a nearly 20-year association with this incredible human being.

Upon entering the office, I was struck by the spartan appearance of the place. Virginia was busy examining patients in the front room; A.M. was busy with patients in the back room. When the three of us finally were introduced to each other, A.M. almost instantly deferred to Virginia, who did virtually all the talking during the interview. Her husband struck me as a rather shy and humble physician who held his wife in the highest professional and personal esteem. At the time, I had no idea of their distinguished backgrounds. To me they were just a couple of people who had a treatment for cancer that interested my editor.

Since I had been a corpsman in the Navy during World War II, I knew more about vaccines and immunity than the average news reporter. Everything the Livingstons told me about their immunologic treatment approach to cancer made sense. In the long conversations I had with Winchell, I had learned that the Runyan fund was also interested in the immunological approach to cancer. But I had no idea that the Fund had given grants to Virginia years earlier.

The rather humble surroundings in which they worked gave me pause. I had no concept of the battles raging for years over the correct approach to cancer treatment. I am sure my questions to the couple must have sounded incredibly sophomoric.

I later learned that the cancer establishment's rejection of Virginia had forced her to ally with "alternative" individuals and groups that sometimes did not fully understand or appreciate what she was trying to accomplish.

Unlike religion, where people can have a choice of beliefs or even non-beliefs, there are only two choices for physicians in medical science. A physician's beliefs can either be orthodox and "accepted"—or unorthodox and totally unaccepted. I am sure that some of Virginia's personal associations with "alternative" cancer therapies must have made her wince on more than one occasion.

I sized up Virginia as a brilliant, kindly, empathetic individual who wore a steel corset under her soft flowing dresses. I was sure if she had been any less powerful in her convictions that she would have been utterly destroyed by the countless lesser people who routinely took every opportunity to shoot arrows at her. Virginia's cancer work was her life—and she never stopped practicing medicine till the day she died.

Some years after meeting "Dr. Virginia," as we called her, I found myself heading a new struggling organization called the Cancer Federation. By that time, A.M. had died and Virginia was married to her fourth husband, physician Owen Wheeler. Owen first met Virginia when he sought treatment as a cancer patient at the Livingston Clinic.

Virginia opened her first clinic in 1969; and the newly named Livingston Medical Center opened in 1971. By 1975 the clinic moved to a brand new building at 3232 Duke Street, in the Point Loma section of San Diego. I remember well my first tour of the beautiful new clinic bustling with activity. I inspected the well equipped laboratory where the blood of cancer patients was examined by use of dark-field microscopes in which Virginia insisted the microbe of cancer could be visualized. I spent an entire day with her and her capable staff, and was especially impressed with the love showered upon her by the patients. While I was there, two famous personalities came into the clinic. One was the actor Lloyd Nolan whose wife was suffering with terminal cancer at the time. Later, he became a life member of the Federation. The other was a powerful California political leader.

Virginia and Owen became enthusiastic supporters of the Cancer Federation. Owen's favorite trick was to hand me a $1,000 check made out to the Federation on his own account, whispering to me to not tell Virginia. On more than one occasion, Virginia wrote a personal check and made me promise not to tell Owen.

The most important gift the Wheelers gave to the Federation was not the money, but rather their many appearances at our annual conferences. In those days their presence drew large crowds to our meetings and attracted considerable media coverage to our events. Six years after our organization began, Virginia co-sponsored a conference with us in San Diego that brought many new and enthusiastic people into the Federation.

When Virginia's fourth husband Owen died in 1988, she was terribly depressed and lonely. But at age 82 she again picked herself up and married a man thirty years younger, which perked her up considerably.

After attending the 60th reunion of the 1930 graduating class at Vassar College, Virginia and her daughter Julie Wagner took off on a European holiday. On June 30, 1990, she died suddenly of a heart attack in Athens, Greece. She was 83 years old.

The obituary in the San Diego *Union Tribune* noted that Virginia was a member of the Daughters of the Revolution and had come to San Diego in 1955 as staff physician at the San Diego Health Association. Later, she was Professor of Microbiology at the University of San Diego and a research associate at the San Diego Biomedical Association. She founded the Livingston Medical Center in 1971.

A Memorial Service honoring her life was held at the Church of Jesus Christ of Latter-day Saints on Torrey Bluff Drive in San Diego on July 12, 1990.

Shortly before her death a study was done comparing her patients with other cancer patients that had undergone "orthodox" treatment. It was concluded that her patients fared as well, or as badly, as those relying exclusively on surgery, radiation or chemotherapy. Not taken into account was the fact that most of Virginia's patients had already been through traditional treatments, and some were given up for dead by the time they got to her clinic.

Cancer is now the leading cause of death for Americans under the age of 85, surpassing deaths from heart disease for the first time. In 2002, the most recent year for which data are available, 476,009 Americans died of cancer, compared to 450,837 who died of heart disease, according to a report issued by the American Cancer Society.

Philosophically, Dr. Virginia added much to the life of the Cancer Federation. Her belief that cancer could be treated by methods designed to improve the immune system's response against the cancer-causing bacteria, did much to shape the direction of the Federation. By 1997, the cancer establishment had "borrowed" many of Virginia's ideas about diet and the use of vaccines to enhance the immune system response.

Virginia Livingston's life was dedicated to the highest ideals and principles of medical science. When the bacterial cause of cancer is finally accepted, as I have no doubt it will, Livingston will finally receive the credit denied her during her lifetime.

She will be heralded as the greatest physician of the twentieth century.

Of that I am sure.

John A. Steinbacher
The Cancer Federation
Banning, California
February 2005
email: info@cancerfed.org

CHAPTER ONE

The Discovery of the Cancer Germ

There is no doubt in my mind that Virginia Livingston was the greatest physician of the twentieth century, even though she was never widely known and is now largely forgotten. Of the people in the cancer establishment who recall her, she is most likely to be remembered as a quack.

I can't write about Livingston without writing about myself because our lives and what we discovered are so closely intertwined. Of all the physicians I have known, she was certainly the smartest, as well as the most controversial, and she influenced me more than all the other doctors put together.

The first half of my life was charted by my father's wish that I become a physician, and as a dutiful son I felt I could not disappoint him. Without his strict guidance, I am sure I would have ended up as a teacher, a musician, an artist, a writer—anything but a doctor. There were too many mysteries, too many unknowns within the human body and that was disconcerting to me. Fortunately I was attracted to dermatology. Skin diseases are something you can see, touch and feel, even though the causes of most skin diseases are also mysterious.

The second half of my life was charted by Livingston, although I think she would have been amazed to discover this. As I write this, it has been exactly a half century since I first entered medical school. When I was a young physician I never dreamed I would play a role in uncovering the infectious germ of cancer.

As a septuagenarian whose life is mostly over, I can now clearly see that Virginia single-handedly influenced the last half of my professional life in ways that continue to astound me.

"Those Little Red Bugs" in Scleroderma

If it were not for a rare skin disease called scleroderma, it is unlikely Virginia and I would have crossed paths. Systemic progressive scleroderma is a horrible and ultimately fatal disease that entombs its victims in rock-hard skin and scars the internal organs.

My introduction to the cancer microbe started innocuously in 1963 as a first-year dermatology resident at the Long Beach VA Hospital in Long Beach, California. While preparing for the weekly Journal Club presentation, I came across a report of some patients who developed deep skin infections after receiving flu shots. The "acid-fast" tuberculosis-type germs causing the problem were identified as a fast-growing, unusual species of acid-fast mycobacteria, known as *Mycobacterium fortuitum*. The source of the mycobacterial infection was never determined.

After reading this interesting report, I decided to take skin biopsies from four of my clinic patients who had inflammatory lesions deep in the fatty portion of the skin. Remarkably, all four "panniculitis" patients showed evidence of acid-fast bacteria in the specially stained microscopic tissue sections, or in stained smears of the biopsy material, or in culture. This was unusual because bacteria were almost never found in reported cases of panniculitis.

My professor J. Walter Wilson, a famous dermatologist and noted expert in fungus infections, was somewhat perplexed because, in his view, I was finding too many patients who were "positive" for acid-fast bacteria. He suggested I get a "control" skin biopsy from Reuben Gomez, a 37-year-old Mexican-American ward patient who was dying with systemic scleroderma. Wilson knew that it would be unlikely to find acid-fast bacteria in Reuben's skin because scleroderma was a disease of unknown etiology—and no bacteria were ever found in that disease.

By choosing Reuben I was set on a path of scientific study from which I could never veer, no matter how hard I tried. It was a path of destiny that led me into the secrets of scleroderma, then into the mysteries of cancer and AIDS, and finally into the origin of life itself.

As I had done with the panniculitis patients, I sent Reuben's skin biopsy specimen to the special tuberculosis (TB) lab where Eugenia Craggs carefully ground-up the tissue, made some skin smears, and planted the material on culture media suitable for growing tuberculosis bacteria.

The acid-fast stain is used to test a specimen for the presence of microorganisms, specifically mycobacteria, the acid-fast bacteria that cause tuberculosis and leprosy. Eugenia placed a dye on the slide and heated it. The tissue cells are stained by the dye. The slide is then washed with an acid solution, and a counter-stain is applied. The bacteria that retain the first dye are acid fast because they resist the acid wash. Bacteria that wash free of the first dye and take the counterstain are nonacid fast.

A few days later she phoned me and said, "This is

Eugenia in TB. I have studied the stained smears, and the specimen on Gomez is positive for acid-fast bacteria."

"That's impossible," I said. "He has scleroderma. There aren't any acid-fast bacteria in scleroderma!" But Eugenia was emphatic. "Well, I don't know anything about scleroderma, but I've been working in TB for years. And I know acid-fast rods when I see them. If you don't believe me, you can come over to the lab and see for yourself."

I asked the pathologist to do a special acid-fast stain on several skin biopsies already taken from Reuben. But I was unable to find any acid-fast bacteria in his slides. I also learned that Reuben had been diagnosed seven years earlier with a mild case of lung TB, which was successfully treated.

After several weeks of incubation, Eugenia grew a microbe from Reuben's skin biopsy tissue, but it was not *Mycobacterium tuberculosis*. What exactly was it? Some of the bacteria were typical rod-shaped and red-stained acid-fast bacteria, but most of the forms were blue-stained round "coccus-like" forms, which were not acid-fast. As the culture aged we observed some forms that were fungus-like and produced long chains and filaments. I had never seen such a peculiar microbe with so many different forms. Eugenia suspected the microbe might be an acid-fast fungus-like bacterium called Nocardia, a closely related species to the Mycobacteria.

In the classification system for bacteria, the acid-fast mycobacteria are closely related to fungi. "Myco" is the Greek work for fungus. For the first half of the twentieth century, only a few species of mycobacteria were important in human and animal disease. The two most common diseases caused by acid-fast bacteria are tuberculosis (caused by *Mycobacterium tuberculosis*), and leprosy (due to *M. leprae*). We were always taught that it was impossible to culture the leprosy bacillus. I later learned from Virginia's microbiologist friend, Eleanor Alexander-Jackson, that she was able to culture strange-looking bacteria from the blood of leprosy patients, but her work was never "accepted."

In the 1960s new species of mycobacteria were being recognized in human disease. This was news to me because we received little training in microbiology in med school. Most physicians don't know much about bacteriology, and most are not trained in microscopic work. However, dermatologists are well-trained in the microscopic appearance of skin diseases, and some even specialize exclusively in the field of dermatopathology.

After many, many hours of studying Reuben's scleroderma tissues (using the highest magnification of the microscope and the oil-immersion lens), I was finally able to detect a few acid-fast rods deep in his skin. The rods were stained bright red and looked just like the typical "acid-fast" rods of the TB and leprosy bacilli. To my disappointment, neither Eugenia nor any of the other microbiologists could precisely identify Reuben's microbe. I quickly learned that microbiology is not the exact science I assumed it was.

I was determined to prove that acid-fast bacteria caused scleroderma, and now I had less than a year before my training would end at the VA. Two more cases were studied and Eugenia found acid-fast bacteria in both. Again, the bacteria were impossible to classify precisely. When my residency ended in 1965, I joined the Dermatology Department at Kaiser-Permanente in Hollywood. I continued to attend weekly conferences at the VA, and to check in on Eugenia's skin cultures. But now her boss resented the time and effort she devoted to my research, and bristled when Eugenia's name appeared (along with Dr. Wilson and Frank Swatek, Professor of Microbiology at Long Beach State College) on our paper on four cases of panniculitis that appeared in the *Archives of Dermatology* in 1966. I was beginning to understand the peculiarities of medical politics, and the fragility of biomedical egos.

When Reuben died in 1967, Lenora, a nurse on the ward, telephoned me. She knew I was desperate to get an autopsy so that I could hunt for acid-fast bacteria in his internal organs. But the family in Arizona refused an autopsy.

Lenora heard my disappointment. "His body was shipped up to East LA yesterday for embalming. Why don't you call the mortician? I'm sure he'll let you take some skin."

I thought she was joking, but she wasn't. "Do you want some skin, or don't you? Why don't you at least try?" I jotted down the address and phone number and thanked her for her bizarre idea. I never would have thought of it myself.

As I drove from Hollywood to the mortuary in East LA, I wondered what madness was overtaking me in my desire to uncover the secrets of scleroderma. Nobody in his right mind did research like this.

The mortician acted like my request was an everyday occurrence. I quickly took several large and deep skin samples. I would never have done such a thing to Reuben while he was alive; it would have been a cruel and savage act. But now he was dead, and Reuben still had something to offer other scleroderma sufferers. I was sure of that.

I sent a skin specimen to the U.S. Public Health

Hospital in Carville, Louisiana, which specializes in the treatment of leprosy (now known as Hansen's disease). Another specimen was sent to Ruth Gordon, a well-known microbiologist at Rutgers University in New Jersey.

Several months later, I got a report from Richard E. Mansfield, M.D., Chief of the Laboratory Branch at Carville, who wrote: "The reason it took so long to get the final report was that a rapid-growing, acid-fast bacterium was cultured from the tissue you sent. We found this to be *Mycobacterium fortuitum*. We have just received confirmation from the National Centers for Communicable Disease (now the CDC), in Atlanta, Georgia. Acid-fast bacteria were found on rare slides."

Dr. Mansfield expressed concern as to whether the tissue might be contaminated, or whether the acid-fast bacteria might have developed after the scleroderma process took hold. Ruth Gordon later wrote that she too had cultured *M. fortuitum*. "We had better luck in recognizing it than some cultures you have sent us." There was no way Reuben's acid-fast bacteria was a contaminant. I was confident it was the same microbe Eugenia had detected a year and a half earlier.

From my work at the VA with Eugenia I learned one important thing: microbes change form. Sometimes they appear one way, sometimes another. And they could fool the experts. The appearance of the microbe depended on what it was fed in the laboratory. And as the culture aged, the germs took on even more unusual forms. In the textbooks of microbiology the classification of organisms was simple and straightforward. But, in reality, it was not that way at all.

By this time I had already developed a reputation as a kooky dermatologist who was frequently finding acid-fast bacteria in diseases "of unknown etiology." Kiddingly, the derm residents at the VA used to greet me with, "Hey, Alan! Found any more little red bugs lately?"

I assumed I was alone in my scleroderma research, but soon I was to discover there were others. Perhaps they could tell me about those strange little red bugs that turned Reuben's skin to stone and finally killed him.

Virginia Livingston and Her Scleroderma Germ

In the spring of 1967 Roy Averill, one of the dermatology residents at the VA, cornered me after the conference and said, "You won't believe this but I was in San Diego this past weekend and I heard a physician being interviewed on the radio. She spoke about finding acid-fast bacteria in scleroderma and cancer. She practices in San Diego. You should have no trouble finding her phone number in the book. Her name is Livingston, Virginia Livingston."

I telephoned. Virginia was delighted to hear about my scleroderma findings, and invited me to San Diego to meet her and her physician husband, A.M.

On my arrival, Virginia deluged me with a pile of published papers she had written with a variety of dermatologists, pathologists, microbiologists, and microscopists. I instantly learned about dozens of other researchers whose work was intimately connected to her research, and to mine.

As an internal medicine resident in New York City, Virginia had special training in detecting the bacteria that cause tuberculosis and leprosy. This training would eventually lead her to discover the germ of cancer.

Years earlier, while examining a school nurse with scleroderma and painful ulcerations of the fingers and nose, Virginia was reminded of leprosy patients she had encountered. Instinctively she took a pin and tested the nurse's skin reaction to pain. Curiously, some scleroderma areas had no feeling.

From the nurse's nasal ulcerations, Virginia scraped some skin tissue onto a microscopic slide and later stained it with an acid-fast dye, just as she had been trained to do with leprosy. She knew if acid-fast bacteria were present, the acid-fast staining procedure would color them red. After placing a thin glass cover-slip on the slide and putting a drop of oil on the slide, she carefully examined the preparation. In the flakes of the scleroderma tissue Livingston found the red-stained, rod-shaped acid-fast microbes that looked exactly like leprosy and TB mycobacteria!

Virginia's discovery was brilliant. But the discovery was the easy part. The hard part would be to get the medical world to accept it. In studying scleroderma, Virginia allied herself to two women: Camille Mermod, a pathologist; and Eva Brodkin, a dermatologist. The three physicians proved that microbes existed in the tissue of scleroderma, and they were successful in culturing bacteria from the skin samples. Virginia injected the scleroderma bacteria into chicks and guinea pigs. The chicks died, and the skin of the guinea pigs hardened like scleroderma. Some guinea pigs even developed cancer. This was very unusual because guinea pigs are highly resistant to cancer.

In July 1947, the *Journal of the Medical Society of New Jersey* published Virginia's paper, "Etiology of scleroderma; A preliminary report," co-authored by Brodkin and Mermod. Five cases of scleroderma were presented. Honoring her maiden and married name at the time, the scleroderma organism was tentatively named "sclerobacillus Wuerthele-Caspe."

The ability of the scleroderma microbe to produce cancer in guinea pigs led Virginia to suspect that a similar microbe might be involved in human cancer. She avidly searched for acid-fast bacteria in various cancer tumor tissue and carefully examined the bacteria that grew from the tumors. By the time the New Jersey journal published her scleroderma report, she had already discovered acid-fast microbes in cancer.

Virginia surrounded herself with talented scientists who aided tremendously in her research. Although 70 years of age, Roy Allen was still an expert microscopist. He possessed a remarkable collection of microscopes, one of which could magnify 2500 times. (Ordinary light microscopes magnify only 1000 times.) He also possessed excellent camera equipment for microphotography.

In, "The microscopy of micro-organisms associated with neoplasms (cancer)" published in the August 1948 issue of *The New York Microscopical Bulletin*, Roy Allen presents illustrations of the cancer microbe and explains how it can be identified in tissue stained with the acid-fast stain. He stressed that the cancer microbe is "pleomorphic," meaning it has more than one appearance. The microbe can be rod-shaped or coccus (round) shaped. The germ can be stained acid-fast (red) or non-acid-fast (blue). The non-acid-fast round coccal forms appear as single, double, or as densely packed round forms. These coccal forms vary in size from 1 micron down to the smallest microscopic size the eye can detect with the microscope (0.2 microns). The microbes live inside the cancer cells (intra-cellular) and outside the cells (extra-cellular). Allen claimed that every pathologist had seen the cancer microbe, but had failed to interpret its true nature.

The tiniest, barely visible forms of the cancer microbe are "filterable" and virus-sized. Viruses are smaller than bacteria; and microbiologists use special laboratory filters to separate viruses and bacteria. Bacterial filters have pore openings which allow the (smaller) viruses to pass through, but not the larger bacteria. Virginia believed the tiny filterable forms of the cancer microbe are related to so-called viruses found in some cancers. These virus forms of the cancer microbe are too small to be seen with the light microscope. However, they can be visualized with the powerful electron microscope which magnifies 60,000 times, or higher.

James Hillier of Princeton used the electron microscope to photograph the virus-sized forms of the cancer microbe at a magnification of 30,000 times. Virginia obtained these pure virus forms by filtering bacterial cultures obtained from cancer tumors.

In order to prove that bacteria originate from these filtered (bacteria-free) cultures, Virginia prepared multiple vials of bacteria-free filtrates from a single cancer microbe culture. Every few days, one of the bottles was opened and the filtrate examined. With the proper growth media and the passage of time, Virginia could induce the cancer bacteria to reappear in the filtered bacteria-free fluid. This was proof that cancer bacteria originated from submicroscopic viruses.

By mid-century Virginia, in collaboration with Roy Allen, bacteriologist John A. Anderson, pathologist Lawrence C. Smith, and microbiologist Eleanor Alexander-Jackson from Cornell University Medical School, had collected enough data to publish their research. In December, 1950, the *American Journal of Medical Sciences* published the group's landmark paper titled "Cultural properties and pathogenicity of certain microorganisms obtained from various proliferative and neoplastic diseases." The eleven-page article contains an electron-microscopic picture of the virus form of the cancer microbe magnified 31,000 times; micro-photographs of the cancer bacteria cultured from the blood and bone marrow of cancer patients; and pictures of diseased lungs and kidneys of animals experimentally infected with the cancer microbe.

The journal provided a classic description of the cancer microbe. "These organisms, which appear primarily as small acid-fast granules in young cultures and which tend to become non-acid-fast in the larger forms present in old cultures, may exhibit a number of types, such as: a) minute filterable granules beyond the limits of visibility of the light microscope; b) larger granules approximately the size of ordinary cocci, readily seen with the light microscope; c) still larger globoidal forms; d) rod-like forms with irregular staining; and e) occasionally globoidal forms which appear to undergo polar budding."

Virginia's discovery of a microbe in cancer should have been heralded as the major medical discovery of the twentieth century. But her controversial research stirred up trouble with powerful people in the cancer establishment. Over the next two decades, the details of her confrontation with the establishment are recorded in her autobiographical book, *Cancer: A New Breakthrough*, published in 1972, now unfortunately out-of-print.

Until her death she could never keep silent about the cancer microbe. The work was too important. She constantly fought the cancer experts, who insisted there was no such thing as bacteria in cancer. Every time she spoke about the cancer microbe, she was inevitably pegged as just another crazy California quack.

I didn't want to get involved in Virginia's conquest of cancer. Even if I wanted to help her, I couldn't. I worked for an establishment institution. I already had a reputation for harboring strange ideas about scleroderma, even though Livingston had discovered acid-fast bacteria in 1947, and even though scientists at the Pasteur Institute in Brussels had also confirmed her findings in 1953.

I had naively thought all this research would change ideas about scleroderma being "a disease of unknown etiology." But, of course, as I would painfully learn, it didn't. Perhaps most importantly, I didn't want to be ostracized professionally like Virginia for antagonizing the medical establishment. She had more courage than I ever thought of having.

Eleanor Alexander-Jackson and Pleomorphism

Where did Virginia learn about pleomorphism, the ability of a microbe to undergo extreme variation in form and size? Certainly this was not taught in medical school. How could she write with such confidence and authority about the cancer microbe when the entire concept was scientific heresy?

In her earliest cancer paper Virginia searched the biomedical literature to prove that microbes did tricks that were unheard of in microbiology. However, as brilliant as she was, there were limits to her ability to explain esoteric microbiologic memorabilia not taught in medical school.

After having met Virginia I soon met her best friend Eleanor who was visiting from New York. Eleanor was the power behind the throne who revealed to Virginia the little-known secrets of bacteriology known to only a few physicians.

I liked Eleanor from the moment I met her. Unlike Virginia, she was reserved and shy. She had a wealth of information to impart about the microbiology of cancer, most of which I didn't understand.

As my frustration with the scleroderma work mounted, I eventually became more interested in Eleanor's research on bacterial pleomorphism. There was no way I could understand scleroderma without learning about pleomorphism. Virginia understood the concept quickly. I was slow; it took years to sink in. When I finally understood it, I knew I had to follow these two women in their quest to unravel the infectious cause of cancer.

Eleanor began studying tuberculosis in 1928, six years before I was born. She quickly discovered unusual growth forms of the tubercle bacillus that were never recorded in the medical books I read. In 1934 she received her doctorate degree in bacteriology. A portion of her thesis describing strange-looking "S" forms of the TB microbe was published in the prestigious *American Review of Tuberculosis.*

Eleanor was a master in detecting and growing TB mycobacteria, and devised a new staining method whereby these bacteria could be identified in tissue specimens. In 1941 she joined the staff of Cornell Medical College as an expert TB microbiologist.

She was intrigued by the "granules," "the coccus-like" and the "globoid" forms of the tubercle bacillus, and could never understand why so few biologists paid attention to these important mutant forms. Eleanor was encouraged, however, by a few researchers who were equally passionate about pleomorphism.

Years after the country doctor Robert Koch discovered the tubercle bacillus in 1882, other microbiologists began to notice "granules" contained within the rod-shaped tuberculosis bacteria. Beginning in 1908 Hans Much wrote extensively about these TB granules and they eventually became known as "Much's granules." The precise nature of the granules remains controversial to this day.

Scientists who experimented with TB granules believed they were part of a "life cycle" of the constantly changing TB germ. In 1910, A. Fontes proved the granules were filterable. Some of these extremely tiny filter-passing forms were too small to be seen microscopically and became known as the TB "virus."

When Fontes injected guinea pigs with these granules they caused immune system disease and tuberculosis. Careful observation revealed some granules enlarging to the size of ordinary-looking cocci; other granules segued into typical acid-fast rods.

Eleanor was the first to write about a slimy "zoo-glear" matrix in which the TB granules formed. Mycobacteriologists also knew that highly virulent and deadly TB germs could degenerate into harmless non-acid-fast cocci and into "diphtheroid" coccobacilli, which looked exactly like common staphylococci and corynebacteria.

All this granule business bored most physicians who couldn't understand why people like Eleanor were wasting time on such matters. But a few dedicated researchers knew the TB granules were extremely important, and might even be involved in the production of cancer!

In 1928, H.C. Sweany claimed that filterable and granular forms of tubercle bacilli could cause Hodgkin's disease, a form of lymphoma cancer. To this day, although a viral infectious agent is suspected in Hodgkin's disease, the role of granular forms of mycobacteria as a cause remains ignored and unexplored.

In 1931, R. Pla y Armengol, a Barcelona scientist, demonstrated that the TB granules were the forms which attacked cells and initiated the TB infection. He also grew pleomorphic TB microbes which looked exactly like fungi! This is similar to what I observed with fungus-like forms isolated from Reuben's scleroderma—and finally identified post-mortem as *Mycobacterium fortuitum*, an "atypical" pleomorphic species of mycobacteria.

In a series of papers published in the 1930s, Ralph Mellon, Lawrence Beinhauer, and L.W. Fisher also declared that mutant TB microbes caused Hodgkin's disease and sarcoidosis—a lung disease resembling tuberculosis and believed to be yet another disease "of unknown etiology." These researchers also proposed a "life cycle" for TB microbes, consisting of forms that were acid-fast and non-acid-fast, and forms that looked exactly like common staphylococci, corynebacteria, and fungi.

For over a decade, Eleanor struggled to prove that the seed of tuberculosis infection is hidden in the granules, in the coccoid forms, and even in the slime of the "zooglear plasmodium." In June 1945, this research was published as "A hitherto undemonstrated zoogleal form of *Mycobacterium tuberculosis*" in the *Annals of the New York Academy of Sciences*.

Soon after discovering acid-fast bacteria in scleroderma, a colleague told Virginia about Eleanor's TB and leprosy research at Cornell. The two women met in 1947 and formed a scientific association and a friendship that lasted over 40 years.

When Eleanor's superiors at Cornell learned she was

collaborating in cancer microbe research with a controversial woman doctor from New Jersey, she was told she might lose her job. During this time she succeeded in culturing pleomorphic acid-fast bacteria from the blood of leprosy patients. Her research was published in 1951 in the *International Journal of Leprosy*.

Few people cared about Alexander-Jackson's contributions to tuberculosis. Like me, they couldn't understand what value it had in detecting bacteria in cancer and scleroderma. Pathologists hunting for TB germs were taught to look *only* for acid-fast *rods*; the rest was unimportant. But when Eleanor began to write about the cancer microbe, powerful people in medical science paid close attention, and some conspired to destroy her career as a research scientist.

"The Three Musketeers" of Cancer Research

During the years 1949-1953, Virginia was able to secure some grant money and opened a laboratory in Newark, New Jersey. The two women were determined to prove that bacteria caused cancer.

Shortly after the lab opened, Irene Corey Diller, Ph.D., joined in the research. Diller was trained as a "cytologist," a specialist in the study of cells. From 1947 until 1971 she was also the editor of *Growth*, a scientific journal devoted to problems of normal and abnormal cell growth. Affiliated with the Department of Chemotherapy at the Institute for Cancer Research in Philadelphia, Irene was assigned the task of determining the effect of chemo-therapeutic agents on cancer cells, as well as normal cells in experimental animals. She primarily worked with laboratory mice and rats, which were specially inbred for cancer tumor research. One day, in her microscopic tumor studies, she noticed a strange-looking body in one of the cancer cells—with a long filament coming out from it. Thinking that the filament looked like a fungus, she began hunting for more odd cancer cells with filaments and found others. She decided to culture the cancerous tissue to see what kind of organism could possibly be infecting her cancer cells.

In culture the microbe looked like a fungus-like bacterium. At the time Irene was unaware that certain bacteria had fungal-like stages in their growth. She certainly did not expect to discover the cause of cancer in the mouse tumors she was investigating, but she believed that if she was working with experimental animal tumors and chemotherapeutic agents, it was important to find out if these tumors were infected with microbes.

In *The Conquest of Cancer (Transcript from a Videotape Program)*, Diller remarks: "These were actual cancers, known and established ones that we use experimentally in mice, and I thought, well, if we are working with tissues that are contaminated or filled with organisms that may change the chemistry of the whole cell, then all of our readings on the cell may need to be revised and we must clear the tissues of these organisms.

So I gave a short abstract at a meeting of the American Association for the Advancement of Science in New York in the Section of Parasitology, and this was picked up by Pat McGrady from the American Cancer Society who had been quite interested in my work. He publicized it a great deal and it got into *Time* and into *Life*, so everybody heard about this, and this is how Virginia first heard about me. Of course, since I was not medically trained, I wasn't reading the medical journals so I didn't know of her earlier work.

Then, when we went into the background of this thing we found that many, many others had found similar organisms, but they called them by all sorts of different names.

Irene attempted to set up a symposium in the early 1950s at the New York Academy of Sciences to present a number of papers on the new research into bacteria as a possible cause of cancer. However, in *The Conquest of Cancer*, Livingston claims Dr. Cornelius P. Rhoads, director of Memorial Sloan-Kettering Cancer Center in New York City, deliberately killed the proposed meeting. Rhoads was Virginia's nemesis. She believed that her finding of an infectious germ in cancer was a threat to his financial interests in promoting cancer chemotherapy.

Prior to the proposed symposium, Irene Diller had accepted several ultraviolet sterilizing lights as a gift from a commercial company for her lab, with no strings attached. But Rhoads used this to declare that the gift was a "commercialization" of her work that made her ineligible to sponsor the meeting at the Academy.

According to Livingston and Addeo's 1984 book, "Dr. Rhoads was committed to chemotherapy, and well he might have been since he was head of chemical warfare during World War II. He tried to turn chemical warfare against the cancer cell within the human body. His big mistake was that he believed the cancer *cell* to be the causative agent of the disease, and not the parasite *within* the cell. To unleash the horrors of chemical warfare and the atomic bomb in the form of chemotherapy and cobalt radiation against the hopeless victims of a microbic disease is illogical. Furthermore, Dr. Rhoads was not content to limit his theories to his own institution but was determined to dictate the research policies of the entire country. At one point he almost succeeded in destroying the basic biological research at the Institute for Cancer Research in Philadelphia and turning the institute into a subservient satellite. Fortunately, he failed."

Despite the cancellation of the meeting, over the following decade Diller's contributions to the microbiology of cancer would be enormous. In more than a dozen published papers, she confirmed Livingston and Alexander-Jackson's microbial findings, and she was confident that the intermittently acid-fast cancer germ was unlike any microbe known to microbiologists.

Nineteen fifty-three was a momentous year for Virginia and Eleanor. In June, the Newark lab team presented their work at an exhibit at the American Medical Association meeting held at the Waldorf-Astoria Hotel in New York City. RCA generously lent an electron microscope which televised the "live" cancer microbe in the blood to the audience. Roy Allen's beautiful color microphotographs and James Hillier's spectacular electron microphotographs were the hit of the AMA convention.

Sensing the threat to orthodox cancer research, the dark forces immediately went into action against the women. The big boys in the medical establishment knew the identification of a cancer microbe could destroy millions of dollars worth of cancer research. The microbe was also a serious threat to the billion-dollar cancer treatment industry. A bacterial "cause" and a possible vaccine "cure" would be financially disastrous for the biomedical business world.

Cancer microbe research has always been the kiss of death for scientists. Again, Virginia thought Cornelius Rhoads put pressure on the press to kill the cancer microbe story. As a result, there was a total press blackout of the popular exhibit at the AMA convention.

In September in Rome, Virginia and Eleanor presented papers at the Sixth International Conference for Microbiology. The conference was a great success and they met other European scientists who had also studied the cancer microbe. Wilhelm von Brehmer, a Berlin scientist, described similar microbes in the blood cells of cancer patients back in the 1930s. Georges Mazet, a French physician, discovered acid-fast bacteria in many different kinds of cancer, including leukemia and Hodgkin's disease, in the 1940s.

While Virginia and Eleanor vacationed in Europe, their enemies succeeded in pulling grant money away from the Newark lab, forcing its closure. Without money there could be no cancer microbe research; and without research the new cancer breakthrough would die a natural death.

Disheartened and disillusioned, and with financial pressures in her family life, Virginia moved to Los Angeles with her husband and daughter to start a new life, and then to San Diego, California, where her father had retired and where her sister lived. Eleanor remained in New York, and Irene Diller continued at the Institute for Cancer Research in Philadelphia.

In 1955 her husband Joseph Caspe died suddenly. In 1957 she married A.M. Livingston, M.D. With the security of a new and successful marriage to a physician, who also had a keen interest in the cancer microbe work, Virginia was definitely on her way up again.

In the 1960s, Eleanor secured some grant money from the National Institutes of Health to study the Rous sarcoma virus, a virus that causes sarcoma cancer in chickens. She proved the Rous virus is actually a filterable form of the cancer microbe. From the cancer microbe, she devised an anti-cancer tumor vaccine that protected healthy chickens against Rous sarcoma disease. As usual, Jackson's research was ignored. Virologists did not want to believe that Rous virus originated from a bacterium.

In 1962, Irene Diller collaborated with Andrew Donnelly and Mary Fisher in a paper titled "Isolation of pleomorphic, acid-fast organisms from several strains of mice," published in *Cancer Research.* They concluded that the tiniest elements of the cancer germ passed through filters designed to hold back bacteria. In addition, the cancer bacteria were found to be closely related to the acid-fast mycobacteria, as well as common non-acid-fast corynebacteria. Could some of these bacteria be infected with so-called "phage viruses," that might make them more pathogenic? Or could these minute, filter-passing forms be "the ultra-fine stages in the life cycle of the bacterium"?

Such questions were not easily answerable. The authors concluded: "In view of the constant association with neoplastic tissues of pleomorphic, intermittently acid-fast bacteria which share antigens in common with Mycobacterium and Corynebacterium, and the fact that the incidence of neoplasia in animals can be experimentally altered by infection with them, it is clear that a study of their role in initiation of disease should be more intensively studied.

"The further fact that some of the strains are both filterable and phage-carrying could offer an explanation of the apparent lack of consistency between the points of view of those who suspect a bacterial and those who suspect a viral induction of neoplasia."

Virginia Livingston suffered a severe heart attack in 1962. Her recovery was slow over the next several years, but it gave her the opportunity to review her past writings and research. In 1965, one of her best papers, an autopsy tissue study of cardiovascular disease co-written by Alexander-Jackson, showed acid-fast microbes in the heart muscle and in the wall of a large artery, as well as in the surrounding connective tissue.

Irene Diller and her biologist husband William wrote a landmark paper in 1965 in the *Transactions of the American Microscopic Society.* Inoculating a large number of healthy mice with bacteria cultured from mice with leukemia, they were able to double the incidence of tumors. In addition, a variety of disease pathology resulted, including the formation of cell "granulomas," abscesses of various internal organs, and degenerative changes in the tissues.

Most importantly, the Dillers showed that cancer germs were able to gain entrance not only into the cell (intra-cellular), but also into the nucleus of the cell. This intra-nuclear invasion meant that cancer microbes could gain access to the genes contained within the nucleus itself. This is similar to what "cancer viruses" do.

In the late 1960s Virginia was able to secure some grants and private donations and allied herself with the University of San Diego. With the support of her husband A.M., she and Eleanor were back in business.

Florence Seibert and the Cancer Microbe

Learning about Irene Diller's research in the early 1960s, Florence Seibert was so impressed that she came out of retirement to help prove that bacteria cause cancer. In the 1920s Seibert devised a method to make intravenous transfusions safe by eliminating contaminating bacteria. Later, as one of the foremost authorities investigating the chemistry and immunology of the acid-fast bacteria that cause tuberculosis, she perfected the skin test for tuberculosis, used worldwide ever since. In 1938, she was awarded the famed Trudeau Medal, the highest prize given for tuberculosis research.

Seibert and her research team isolated bacteria from every tumor and every acute leukemic blood they studied, proving these acid-fast and TB-like cancer microbes were not laboratory contaminants.

In her autobiography, *Pebbles on the Hill of a Scientist*, published privately in 1968, she wrote: "One of the most interesting properties of these bacteria is their great pleomorphism [ability to change form]. For example, they readily change their shape from round cocci, to elongated rods, and even to thread-like filaments, depending upon what medium they grow on and how long they grow. This may be one of the reasons why they have been overlooked or considered to be heterogeneous contaminants. Even more interesting than this is the fact that these bacteria have a filterable form in their life cycle; that is, they can become so small they pass through bacterial filters which hold back bacteria. This is what viruses do, and is one of the main criteria of a virus, separating them from bacteria. But the viruses also will not live on artificial media like these bacteria do. They need body tissue to grow on. Our filterable form, however, can be recovered again on ordinary artificial bacterial media, and will grow on these. This should interest the virus workers very much and should cause them to ask themselves how many of the viruses may not be filterable forms of our bacteria."

After 30 years of studying the acid-fast bacteria that cause tuberculosis, Seibert knew that the discovery of a pleomorphic and acid-fast microbe in cancer was tremendously important. She fervently believed that knowledge of this microbe would be instrumental in developing a possible vaccine, as well as an effective antibiotic therapy against cancer.

In *Pebbles*, she writes: "It is very difficult to understand the lack of interest, instead of great enthusiasm, that should follow such results, a lack of certainty not in the tradition of good science. The contrast between the progress made in tuberculosis, where we know the cause, where we have good general diagnostic tests, where we have a vaccine and effective antibiotic controls, and that made in cancer with the millions invested, is very striking. Some dedicated scientists should indeed find it rewarding to confirm or deny these painstaking and time-consuming experiments, for the sake of establishing the first necessary step in the important problem of the etiology of cancer."

Like the other women, Seibert observed the virus-like forms of the cancer microbe within the nucleus of the cancer cells. She theorized this infection could disrupt and transform nuclear genetic material that could lead to malignant change. Even though cancer microbes might appear to be simple and common microbes, their ability to infiltrate the nucleus of cells meant they were far from harmless.

I sent one of my scleroderma papers to Irene Diller. She responded in a letter, dated Oct 16, 1967. "Thank you for the reprint of your interesting paper on organisms from scleroderma. They look very much like our own isolates. Perhaps we are deluding ourselves, but I don't see how these organisms can be so consistently associated with disease and be unrelated to etiology, even if only as secondary vectors for viruses. Keep up your courage; it is true that this is a frustrating field, but one cannot let it go, as it seems so much more promising than other leads in cancer."

The New York Academy of Sciences Meeting in 1969

Virginia's critics labeled her a quack because she saw cancer bacteria that cancer experts would not or could not see. And she sought to treat cancer patients with a vaccine made to stimulate the immune system against a cancer germ infection. Her microbe could appear sometimes as a common staphylococcus, sometimes as a "diphtheroid" or coccobacilli, or as a fungus, or as an invisible "virus" that could not be detected microscopically. *The cancer microbe violated the established laws of microbiology!*

In 1969, the cancer microbiologists were finally given an opportunity to speak at a conference titled "Unusual Isolates From Clinical Material." At the meeting sponsored by the New York Academy of Sciences, Virginia, Eleanor, Irene, Florence, and a host of other researchers all spoke about their experiences with pleomorphic bacteria in cancer. The proceedings are officially recorded in *The Annals of the New York Academy of Sciences* (Volume 174; 1970), an indispensable document for students of the microbiology of cancer.

In the previous decade, Virginia had renamed the cancer germ *Mycobacterium tumefasciens humanis*, the human strain. Later, she was asked to re-classify it into a separate group because the microbe differed in some ways from mycobacteria. At the meeting, Virginia and Eleanor decided to give the cancer microbe a new classification and characterization. Henceforth it would be known as

Progenitor cryptocides; and classified in the order Acti-nomycetales, the family Progenitoraceae, and the genus *Cryptocides* (in Greek meaning, "hidden killer").

The new name, *P. cryptocides*, was undoubtedly yet another reason for microbiologists and colleagues to attack the women for having the audacity to classify a microbe that did not even exist and was not recognized by the scientific community.

The provocative papers presented at the prestigious Academy should have caused a stir. But with these four women slowly closing in on the infectious cause of cancer, funds from previous supporters (such as the American Cancer Society) suddenly dried up again.

It was obvious the medical establishment did not want to uncover an infectious agent in cancer. The identification of such a germ would destroy established cancer research and pose a severe threat to the radiation and chemotherapy business. Cancer virologists would look like fools if their viruses were discovered to actually be small forms of bacteria. In short, the cure for cancer did not include a cancer germ in the scenario.

For more than a half-century all aspects of cancer microbe research had been suppressed by medical science. Now with the four women zeroing in on the cause of cancer, it was imperative that the suppression continue permanently.

CHAPTER TWO

The History of the Cancer Germ

No one in medical history ever tried harder than Virginia Livingston to convince a disinterested medical establishment that bacteria were the cause of cancer. She wrote numerous papers in reputable medical journals. She wrote several books on the subject, hosted many conferences, did radio talk shows, spoke at cancer conventions—and she ran a clinic devoted to the treatment of cancer for two decades. She never claimed to be the first to discover the cancer germ, but she was the first to relate the microbe to the mycobacteria, and was the first to discover that the acid-fast stain was the key to revealing its identity, not only in culture but in the cancerous tissue as well. Unlike some famous scientists of today, she never failed to give credit to scientists who went before her and who contributed greatly to the microbiology of cancer.

William Russell and the "Cancer Parasite"

In my reading and research I learned that "the parasite of cancer" was seriously discussed at the close of the nineteenth century by top-notch scientists of that era.

When bacteria were first discovered in tuberculosis and other infectious diseases, it was thought they might also be involved in cancer. In 1890, the distinguished pathologist William Russell (1852-1940) first reported "cancer parasites" in cancer tissue that was specially stained with carbol fuchsin, a red dye. The "parasite" was found inside and outside the cells. The smallest forms were barely visible microscopically; and the largest parasites were as large as red blood cells. Russell also found "parasites" in tuberculosis, syphilis, and skin ulcers.

Other scientists quickly disputed his findings, but Russell's pleomorphic "parasites" are well known to modern day pathologists as "Russell bodies." The bodies are believed to be non-microbial "immunoglobulins" (protein substances) formed within blood "plasma cells." In my book *The Cancer Microbe* (1990), Russell bodies are shown in a lymph node of Hodgkin's disease. It is my belief that the largest Russell bodies actually represent "giant L forms" of "cell-wall-deficient bacteria," also known to microbiologists as "large bodies."

After three years of cancer research at the New York State Pathological Laboratory of the University of Buffalo, Harvey Gaylord confirmed Russell's research in a 36-page report titled "The protozoon of cancer," published in May 1901, in the *American Journal of the Medical Sciences*. Gaylord found the variably sized round forms characteristic of Russell bodies in every cancer he examined. Some large spherical bodies were four times the diameter of a leukocyte (white blood cell). Thus, some of the bodies that Gaylord observed attained the amazing size of around 50 microns in diameter. In addition, he found evidence of internal segmentation within the larger bodies "after the manner recognized in malarial parasites." The tiniest forms appeared the size of ordinary staphylococci.

By the early part of the twentieth century, the top cancer experts rejected the cancer parasite as the cause of cancer. The highly influential American pathologist James Ewing, in his widely read textbook, *Neoplastic Diseases*

(1919), wrote that "few competent observers consider it (the parasitic theory) as a possible explanation in cancer." In Ewing's view, cancer did not act like an infection. Therefore, microbes could not possibly cause cancer. He concluded, "The general facts of the genesis of tumors are strongly against the possibility of a parasitic origin." As a result, few doctors dared to contradict Ewing's dogma by continuing the search for a cancer germ.

Young, Nuzum, and Scott's Cancer "Coccus"

James Young, an obstetrician from Scotland, refused to be intimidated by Ewing or anyone else. He repeatedly grew pleomorphic bacteria from breast, uterine and genital cancer, and from cancerous lymph nodes. The microbe had a specific "life cycle" with a "spore stage" comprised of exceedingly tiny and barely visible spores. In laboratory culture the spores transformed into larger coccoid forms, yeast-like forms, and rods. In a 1921 paper, Young claimed the cancer parasite was related to common bacteria which are found everywhere in nature. Young's cancer microbe met with a hostile reception.

During the 1920s, Chicago physician John Nuzum consistently cultured a pleomorphic coccus from breast cancer in mice, and from human breast cancer. Some of the cocci were tiny virus-sized forms which easily passed through a filter designed to hold back bacteria.

In 1925, *Northwest Medicine* published two papers by Montana surgeon Michael Scott who learned about the cancer microbe in T. J. Glover's lab in 1921. Scott's microbe was strikingly similar to Young's. Scott believed cancer was an infection like tuberculosis, and he devised a promising vaccine that cured some hopeless cancer patients. However, his treatment methods were quickly suppressed by the medical establishment. According to Robert Netterberg and Robert Taylor's *The Cancer Conspiracy* (1981), Scott became "a forgotten man," who died in California in 1967, "hopeful to the end."

In 1929, the Stearns and B. F. Sturdivant, microbiologists in Pasadena, California, repeatedly isolated pleomorphic bacteria from cancer tumors. They could not classify the microbe because of its highly complex growth forms, which included tiny and large cocci, rods, and fungal forms. A year later, Glover was the first to consistently isolate cancer microbes from the blood of cancer patients. "Old" laboratory cultures of the microbe transformed into "spore bearing bacilli" and fungi with large "spore sacs."

The "Granules" in Scleroderma

While Livingston and her women colleagues were telling the world about the cancer microbe, I was content to study scleroderma, assuming that some other dermatologist or pathologist would surely find acid-fast bacteria, and culture pleomorphic bacteria from scleroderma skin, as I had done. Forty years later there is still no additional confirmation.

The problem, of course, was that finding typical acid-fast rods that looked exactly like the tuberculosis mycobacteria could consume hours and hours of often fruitless time spent peering into a microscope. It is not likely that a skeptical physician would want to attempt this. It is possible to detect acid-fast bacteria in scleroderma, but hunting for them was as time-consuming and frustrating as looking for four-leaf clovers.

Virginia kept prodding me to get involved in cancer

research, but she was becoming more and more notorious, particularly for her use of "autogenous" vaccines made from the patient's own *Progenitor cryptocides.*

By the late 1970s my scleroderma research had stalled, but it was revived by a patient named Abe Greenstein who had a very unusual form of scleroderma. When he came to my office he said, "My dermatologist tells me you have studied scleroderma. He says you know what causes it." I must say my ego got a boost when I heard that.

He insisted I study his skin and offered me as many skin biopsy samples as I needed. Luckily and rather quickly I was able to detect a few typical acid-fast rods in his skin biopsy tissue. My faith in my research was miraculously restored, and from that moment my search for bacteria resumed with a frenzy.

When I first met Virginia in 1967, she introduced me to Dan Kelso, a Los Angeles bacteriologist, who became a good friend and who has been responsible for growing most of the microbes cultured from my scleroderma and cancer patients since that time.

When Dan repeatedly cultured microbes from Abe that looked like common staphylococci and common coccobacilli (corynebacteria, "diphtheroids"), I was extremely disappointed. Where were the acid-fast rods? Finally, on a smear from a 13-day culture we identified some acid-fast bacteria that looked exactly like the rod forms of tuberculosis-type microbes! Abe's unusual scleroderma case and microbiological findings were published in the *Archives of Dermatology* in 1980.

It is said that people see only what they are looking for; and that may be why the microbiology of cancer is so difficult to comprehend for most physicians. However, once you know how to stain the microbe and know what it looks like—it is found in many diseases. On the other hand, if you don't believe it exists—it is nowhere to be found. In my publications I have always shown pictures of these bacteria in various disease states, but it is still claimed that cancer microbes do not exist. Truly a surreal situation!

After studying scleroderma tissue for over a decade, I finally began to pay serious attention to the tissue "granules" and the round "coccoid forms" that I had seen, but previously ignored. As Sherlock Holmes might have said, "Alan, You see but you do not observe." Virginia and Eleanor insisted the granules and coccoid forms were actual forms of the microbe; but the expert pathologists and dermatologists insisted they were merely "mast cell granules" or some sort of cell debris or extraneous stain deposit of no consequence. How could I convince them that the "granules" were microbes?

Back in 1948, Roy M. Allen wrote in "The microscopy of micro-organisms associated with neoplasms" in the New York Microscopic Society Bulletin, that "it is probable that these organisms have been seen and noted by practically every pathologist, but interpreted as eosinophilic [pink] granules. Hence their true nature was not recognized. Only the Ziehl-Neelsen technique [acid-fast stain] reveals their true nature."

Mast cells have a nucleus, but there were scattered granular and coccoid forms in the scleroderma tissue with no cell nucleus in sight. Of course, the pathologists had no knowledge of, or interest in, the "granular" microbes we cultured from scleroderma. They were not trained in examining bacterial cultures; that was the domain of the bacteriologist. But the more I studied and "observed" the round bacterial forms that we grew in the lab and compared them to what was observed in tissue, the more I realized that some of what we grew in the lab was identical to what I could see in the acid-fast tissue sections prepared by the pathology department.

When Eleanor strongly recommended that I read microbiologist Lida Mattman's *Cell Wall Deficient Forms* (1974), I was stunned to learn that tuberculosis-type microbes exist in many forms, none of which I had ever been taught in medical school. Lida wrote about numerous researchers who described a "life cycle" for mycobacteria that included virus-size forms, bacterial forms, and giant forms known as "large bodies." I also learned that the tubercle bacillus and other bacteria can grow into very large structures, attaining the size of red blood cells, or even larger!

I was later able to identify some "large bodies" in cancer tissue, AIDS, scleroderma, and other diseases. I was sure these "large body" forms of bacteria were exactly what Russell had observed and described as the pleomorphic "parasite of cancer" back in the late nineteenth century. According to Mattman, "Much's granules" and Eleanor's "zooglear forms" were all part of the life cycle of tuberculosis germs. I was delighted to finally meet Lida in person, and to learn she was a big fan of Eleanor's research. In a chapter in her book titled, *Microbes and Malignancy*, I learned about the research of dozens of other microbiologists who believed bacteria cause cancer. A second edition of *Cell Wall Deficient Forms; Stealth Pathogens* was published in 1993, and is a superb source of reference material on the microbiology of cancer and the variability and pleomorphism of bacteria.

The various forms and sizes and shapes of the TB

microbe are all the result of changes in the "cell wall" of the microbe. I concluded that the granular and the round coccoid forms of the scleroderma microbe had the characteristics of Mattman's so-called "cell-wall-deficient forms" (also known as "L-forms," "mycoplasma" and "PPLO-like" microbes). The editors of the *Archives of Dermatology* kindly allowed me to present these revolutionary ideas in our paper describing Abe's rare case of "nodular scleroderma" and the pleomorphic bacteria associated with his disease.

To strengthen my claims of a bacterial cause of scleroderma, Florence Seibert advised me to study autopsied cases to determine if similar microbes could be identified in the affected internal organs. With the help of a pathologist, I was able to identify pleomorphic bacteria in the heart, lungs, kidneys, adrenal glands, and connective tissue of a woman who died of systemic scleroderma. Details of this autopsied case were published in *Dermatologica* in 1980, along with various photos of the microbes in the internal organs.

The Cancer Microbe and its Growth Hormone

Virginia presented one of her greatest and most original discoveries to the scientific world in 1974 in the *Transactions of the New York Academy of Sciences* ("Some cultural, immunological, and biochemical properties of *Progenitor cryptocides*"). In *The Conquest of Cancer* she writes that the cancer germ secretes a human and mammalian hormone called choriogonadotropin hormone (CG). This is important because CG is a hormone necessary for life itself to begin. According to Livingston, "all reproductive life, whether of the fetus *in utero* or of the cancer cell, is controlled by CG."

CG is present in the sperm: "When the sperm enters the ovum (egg), the secretion of CG by the *P. cryptocides* envelops the new life (zygote) so that the mother's immune system does not reject the fetus. The placenta is coated with CG, protecting the fetus from the mother's immune system, and the mother from invasion by the fetal cells [which is 'foreign' to the mother because half the genetic material belongs to the father]. Therefore, when one considers that the *P. cryptocides* is carried by human sperm and is required for new life to evolve and survive (because it is the source of CG), it is not difficult to understand how this potentially killing but also reparative microbe exists in all human cells. However, the microbe remains dormant until our immune systems become so weak as to let it gain a foothold, at which time its secretion of CG allows a tumor to grow. Every tumor has large amounts of uncontrolled proliferation."

Ron Falcone hosts a website devoted exclusively to research pertaining to cancer bacteria. There is much up-to-date information and research on human choriogonadotropin hormone (HCG). "Livingston's HCG findings have potentially solved one of the greatest medical mysteries of all time, i.e. how cancer cells grow unchecked, without attack by the immune system. What does HCG and the human fetus have to do with cancer and bacteria? According to Livingston, malignant tumors are like perverse human fetuses whose intent are to grow and become 'full adults' (which, of course, they can never become), and like the fetus, tumors use HCG to fend off attack from the immune system. Not only do bacteria play a possible role in triggering the cancer process, but they also help in the production of HCG. It may very well be that

Livingston will one day be recognized as the first scientist to provide a solution to the age-old puzzle of how cancer cells escape attack by the immune system."

Falcone also says HCG has been found to be a universal cancer marker, and cancer bacteria have been shown to produce HCG in significant amounts. This means that cancer bacteria may be used to create vaccines that target HCG molecules on the cancer cell, opening a path to destruction of cancer by the immune system. Such vaccines might be used in both the treatment and prevention of cancer. Therapies which do not address the issue of cancer bacteria and HCG may not be successful in curing the disease. For example, toxic chemotherapy is designed to kill malignant cells by inhibiting DNA synthesis. But, as a consequence, it also destroys healthy cells and compromises the immune system. In addition, many recent "breakthroughs" involving monoclonal antibodies, interleukins, tumor-necrosis factors, gene therapies, angiogenesis inhibitors, etc. have only shown partial success. "Could these therapies be significantly bolstered with a revised therapeutic approach as suggested by the research outlined in this website?" Falcone asks.

In her letters to me, Florence Seibert expressed doubt as to whether all bacteria cultured from cancer were a specific organism, as Virginia and Eleanor believed. Some of Seibert's microbes did not belong to a single type of bacteria. She wanted to keep an open mind on this. In a letter dated January 31, 1978, she noted that bacteria can incorporate some human genes for making various hormones such as insulin and choriogonadotropin hormone. So she felt the reverse could be true also. That bacteria could also incorporate human genes into their own cells. In addition, there are "phage" viruses that infect bacteria,

so-called "bacteriophages." Seibert believed a virus infecting a bacterium could change its genetic structure and growth
pattern, and could make the bacterium more pathogenic.

The Sarcoidosis Connection to Cancer

In the late 1970s I was awarded a yearly grant of several
thousand dollars to determine whether acid-fast bacteria
might play a role in certain skin diseases. In 1977 I studied two women with areas of "pseudoscleroderma" con-
fined to the lower leg. The patients did not have scleroderma, but had scleroderma-like hardening of the leg skin,
which was inflamed and painful. I discovered acid-fast
microbes and "large bodies" in these cases, which were
reported in the *Archives of Dermatology* in 1979.

I also studied Georgette, another woman with
pseudoscleroderma, who also had "sarcoidosis." This
inflammatory disease can affect many organs of the body,
most commonly the lungs. Lung sarcoidosis closely
resembles tuberculosis. Although a number of researchers
have claimed sarcoidosis is an infectious bacterial disease,
it is generally believed that the disease is not caused by
microbes. The disease is considered "of unknown
etiology." I could never understand these discrepancies
in science. It just is. As someone who has discovered
bacteria in a number of diseases "of unknown etiology, "
it is very frustrating to have your published research
neither denied nor confirmed nor cited, only ignored by
the "experts" in the field. Of course, this is a common
complaint of all cancer microbe researchers.

A biopsy of Georgette's scleroderma-like leg lesion
was performed and, when I received the pathologist's
report diagnosing the case as sarcoidosis, I was totally

confused. I had never observed scleroderma changes in the skin "mixed" with the pathologic "granulomatous" inflammatory changes of sarcoid.

Georgette was born in 1924. In the early 1970s she went blind due to "uveitis." In 1975, two years before she became my patient, a surgeon removed one of her lungs and some lymph nodes because of suspected lung cancer. After the tissue was examined, the pathologist discovered that she had sarcoid, not cancer. The lab also tested for TB, but no mycobacteria could be found. I requested that I be allowed to study the stored lung and lymph node tissue. Using the acid-fast stain, I was able to detect pleomorphic bacteria in the specimens.

Although microbes are not recognized in sarcoidosis, I detected pleomorphic microbes in every patient I studied with that disease. In reading Mattman's book, I came across references to the experiments of Dr. C. Xalabarder at the Francisco Moragas Antituberculosis Institute in Barcelona, Spain. He experimentally produced sarcoidosis in animals by injecting them with cell-wall-deficient forms of TB bacteria that he cultured from "inactive" TB cases. On the basis of his extensive research (most of which is recorded in Spanish), Xalabarder concluded that sarcoidosis is a form of tuberculosis caused by pleomorphic TB microbes!

For decades pathologists have also recognized a peculiar relationship between sarcoid and cancer (especially lymphoma cancer). For example, tissue pathologic changes resembling sarcoid have been found in lymph nodes that drain cancer tissue.

One of my elderly patients had several skin lesions of sarcoid, but showed no signs of lung disease or cancer. However, a year and a half later she began to develop night sweats, fever and chills, and swollen lymph nodes. One of the enlarged nodes was diagnosed as lymphoma cancer. Photographs of the acid-fast microbes I detected in her skin and cancerous lymph node were published in the *International Journal of Dermatology* in 1982.

After I learned the strange link between sarcoid and cancer, it was inevitable that I would begin to study cancer. For years I put off studying cancer because I didn't want to be controversial like Virginia. The die was cast when a young mother with four young children sought my advice about some small lumps which had recently appeared on her chest. When Alice lowered the sheet covering her chest, I saw the scars and the absence of breasts. I took two skin biopsies, one for the pathologist, the other for Dan Kelso to culture for bacteria.

The pathologist's report showed metastasis of the breast cancer to the skin. With the spread to the skin, Alice did not have much more time to live. Within a few months the cancer spread to her lungs and liver. Dan cultured the cancer microbe, and I discovered the microbe in her stored breast tissue and in her skin samples. Our paper, "Microbial findings in cancer of the breast and in their metastases to the skin," was published in the *Journal of the Dermatologic Surgery and Oncology* in 1981. It was one of the proudest days of my life.

I was forty-six years old and I was beginning to understand my purpose in life, and why I was different from the rest. I knew I had the courage to join Virginia in showing the cancer microbe to the world. I could no longer remain silent.

And I no longer gave a damn about the consequences.

Acid-Fast Bacteria in Cancer Tissue

In the late 1970s and early 1980s, when I became fully confident that the cancer germ in tissue was primarily in the granular, coccoid, and Russell body form, my cancer microbe research proceeded by leaps and bounds. I still was receiving a small yearly grant, which helped the pathology department recoup some of the costs of the special stains, and I could afford to pay Dan Kelso for culturing my skin biopsy specimens, and for the costs of the microphotography.

Between 1980 and 1986, I was able to get papers published showing the microbe in breast cancer, lymphoma, Hodgkin's disease, pre-AIDS Kaposi's sarcoma, as well as in non-cancerous diseases like sarcoidosis, scleredema and vasculitis, and in autopsied cases of scleroderma and lupus erythematosus. These were the early years of the AIDS epidemic. Prior to the discovery of HIV, I showed that the cancer microbe was operative in the swollen lymph nodes of AIDS, in AIDS-related Kaposi's sarcoma, in an AIDS-related immunoblastic sarcoma, and disseminated throughout the body in an autopsied case of AIDS.

In June of 1984, the same year that HIV was discovered, my first book, *AIDS: The Mystery and the Solution,* was published. It was my belief that the cancer microbe played an important part in the development of full-blown AIDS, and numerous pictures of the cancer microbe were presented in AIDS-damaged tissue.

While my book was on the press, Virginia's book *The Conquest of Cancer*, co-written by Ed Addeo, was published and caused quite a stir. Prior to publication, Virginia had asked me for a blurb to be printed on the back cover. Naturally I consented, and when the blurb was published in the *Los Angeles Times* in a book advertisement, all hell broke lose at the clinic. Below my quote was printed my name and association with The Southern California Permanente Medical Group (part of Kaiser Permanente). Before I knew it I was bombarded with memos from the head of the Group, demanding to know why I was associating myself with this quack doctor, and causing untold embarrassment to the organization. When it was discovered that I also had a book on AIDS on the press, the top brass hit the roof.

I had thought I was entitled to free speech, but the Group thought differently. Fortunately, I had retained a literary lawyer who met with their lawyers, and it was agreed I could publish the book, but all reference to Kaiser Permanente had to be expunged from the book.

Now I felt the intense pressure and power of medical politics directed against me. From that point on it was downhill for my research and my yearly small grant. When I was directed to meet with a statistician to discuss my research, I knew I was being set-up for a fall. When he asked if I intended to find cancer microbes in every disease I studied, I knew it was the end of my research.

Ironically, no one really seemed to care about the finding of bacteria in cancer anyway. I never received any accolades for having so many papers published in medical journals in such a short time. In my view, physicians were totally clueless when it came to any notion that bacteria could be routinely observed and photographed in cancer.

Robert Gallo Versus Virginia Livingston

On April 6, 1984, following the publication of *The Conquest of Cancer*, an unflattering article appeared in the *Los Angeles Times,* titled "New 'Cure' for Cancer Stirs Controversy; Livingston-Wheeler contends disease is caused by bacteria." The story included a vicious attack by Robert Gallo of the National Cancer Institute.

At this time and up to the present, Gallo was the most famous virologist in the world for his AIDS research. His official "discovery" of HIV (the human immunodeficiency virus) as the cause of AIDS was hailed in the world media two weeks later on April 23rd. In the *Times* piece, Gallo expressed frustration that Livingston had not published anything in a legitimate medical journal for the past decade, thus not making available any scientific data to substantiate her claim. He said, "It makes me uncomfortable because, while the idea that cancer is a bacterially caused disorder has no apparent scientific basis, scientists haven't been given enough information on Livingston-Wheeler's work to know what to make of her claims, or where to begin in refuting them." In a rant, he declared: "What is going on in this country? This is insanity! She can have her theories and what can I say? I don't know anything to support it. I can't see any basis and I don't know what to say or what analogy to give you."

Virginia's private response was that Gallo should spend more time reviewing the scientific literature, instead of making unsubstantiated accusations about her work to the press.

I was the only physician who came to her defense in the *Times* article, which further inflamed the head physician at Kaiser Permanente who accused me in a nasty memo of associating with "that quack doctor." When asked by the *Times* why there were so few adherents of her ideas, I said, "I think it's because doctors have become absolutely convinced there is no microbe (cause) in cancer. If you ask them why, they say it's because that's what they learned in medical school. I know it does sound somewhat insane, but, I too, keep seeing things that look like microbes under the microscope. I think it's a shame that more people are not seeing them. Remember, microbes were around for centuries before doctors decided they were important in disease."

Virginia and Eleanor's research had long posed a threat not only to powerful physicians in the cancer establishment, but also to virologists who had taken over cancer research in the early 1970s as a result of Richard Nixon's so-called War on Cancer. When the genetic code was broken in the 1950s, virologists took a second look at Peyton Rous's transmissible chicken sarcoma virus that he discovered in 1911. After being ignored for decades, Rous's virus became used widely in cancer virus research and formed the basic framework of modern day virology and genetic engineering.

Rous never named his RNA chicken sarcoma virus "a virus," but rather "a filterable transmissible agent." Like the germ of cancer, the "agent" passed through a filter designed to hold back bacteria and cells. His original 1911 paper in *JAMA* is titled "Transmission of a new malignant growth by means of a *cell-free filtrate*."

Rous contracted lymph node tuberculosis as a medical student, and later developed pulmonary TB during his postgraduate training as a pathologist. Virginia and Eleanor had many meetings with Rous, who won the Nobel Prize in medicine in 1966 at the age of 87 for the work he did decades earlier.

In 1966 Jackson demonstrated in *Growth* that the Rous virus was actually a filterable virus-sized form of the cancer microbe ("Mycoplasma [PPLO] isolated from Rous sarcoma virus"). In 1970 another of her papers was published in the *Annals of the New York Academy of Sciences* that demonstrated (by use of spectograms obtained with the ultraviolet spectogramic microscope) that the RNA Rous sarcoma agent contained traces of DNA—thus indicating the Rous "virus" was essentially related to bacteria that Eleanor had consistently isolated from cancer.

Along with Gallo, the *Times* reporter Allan Parachini interviewed Dr. Ludwig Gross, author of one of the leading texts on cancer viruses. "The whole thing doesn't make any sense," said Gross, who knew Rous personally before Rous died in 1990. "There has never been any doubt that Rous was onto the viral theory of cancer—not a bacterial one."

In my files, I have a copy of a letter dated September 4, 1967, that was sent to Eleanor and signed by Rous. It reads, "Dear Doctor Alexander-Jackson: The pressure upon me since the Nobel Prize has been such that only now have I read with close attention the paper about your PPLO. Your facts make my mind do less than swim, they almost submerge it! With what complexities is the RSV [Rous sarcoma virus] now beset. I'm glad to have quitted it while it was simple. With appreciation of your kind note, Sincerely, Peyton Rous, M.D."

The relationship between cancer in chickens and the Rous agent was part of the reason Virginia's so called "anti-cancer" diet recommended the avoidance of chicken and eggs. This was considered absolute nonsense by her detractors but based on her bacterial research, she believed strongly that chickens were not healthy for cancer patients to eat. According to Livingston, it was hard enough eradicating the build-up of their cancer microbes. Therefore, why add more cancer bacteria to the diet by ingesting diseased and poorly processed chicken.

After his "discovery" of HIV, Gallo was immediately challenged by Luc Montagnier and researchers at the Pasteur Institute in Paris, who claimed Gallo had stolen the AIDS virus from them and had incorporated the French discovery into his own research—and then had the arrogance to present the virus to the world as Gallo's own discovery. The sordid affair resulted in a highly publicized lawsuit, which was finally settled in 1987 through the interventions of president Ronald Reagan and the French premier. Details of this research scandal are chronicled in Pulitzer Prize-winning author John Crewsdon's *Science Fictions: A Scientific Mystery, A Massive Cover-Up, and the Dark Legacy of Robert Gallo* (2002).

Virginia Livingston and Man-Made AIDS

For five years prior to the discovery of HIV, I had studied bacteria in Kaposi's sarcoma, the skin tumor that would be called the "gay cancer" of AIDS. I couldn't understand why scientists and colleagues were paying no attention to the acid-fast bacteria I reported in this disease, particularly during the early years of the epidemic when the cause of AIDS and KS was unknown.

When Robert Gallo and Luc Montagnier both declared themselves the discoverers of HIV, I wondered why they always failed to mention bacteria in this disease. As a result, I always felt there was something amiss in the science and the politics surrounding AIDS. And I was saddened by the loss of many friends and patients from this awful disease during this period.

Some people who read Virginia's writings were irked about her thoughts on human sexuality, particularly her view suggesting that promiscuity could lead to cancer and transfer of cancer-causing bacteria. In her 1972 book, she advised: "Be careful of your personal contacts. Do not have physical relations except with your mate. Promiscuity leads to venereal disease, exposure to cancer, and is sinful."

This also startled some readers because cancer was known to be non-contagious; and Virginia was saying that promiscuity could somehow lead to cancer, a rather far-out belief at the time. However, over the past two decades it has become increasingly clear that the sexually transmitted "herpes-2 virus" can lead to cervical cancer. And certainly with HIV infection and the intense fear surrounding AIDS, Virginia's once controversial sexual admonitions now make perfect sense.

I also wondered if perhaps the sexual revolution of the 60s and 70s and the widespread use of antibiotics for venereal disease might have transformed the cancer microbe into a more virulent kind of bacteria that might be more easily transmitted between people, particularly people who were immunosuppressed or on drugs, or both. I wrote about this in *AIDS: The Mystery and the Solution.*

It was hard for me to imagine that my friendship with Virginia could get me into any more hot water than it already had. But in 1986 she was again responsible for plunging me into a nightmare from which I have never fully recovered.

I remember distinctly the early morning phone call in August 1986 that started it all. At age 79, Virginia was still a human dynamo, working full time at the cancer clinic she founded in 1969, and still proclaiming (to anyone that would listen) that the cancer germ caused cancer.

After a brief hello, Virginia quickly got to the point. "Alan, I have just heard the most dreadful thing. I've been in touch with a medical doctor in Los Angeles, and he says the whole AIDS virus thing was deliberately engineered."

My mind was racing to keep up with Virginia. What in God's name was she talking about? Despite my objections, she insisted: "I want you to come down to San Diego this weekend to meet the doctor. His name is Robert Strecker. Some other doctors will be here too. You must come."

When I arrived with my partner Frank, my uneasiness settled once we found ourselves pleasantly chatting with an interesting group of people in the huge, exquisitely furnished living room of Virginia and Owen Wheeler's spectacular hilltop home, overlooking the Pacific Ocean in La Jolla.

Robert Strecker was an excellent researcher and although I was not immediately convinced of his accusations, I began a serious study of the theory that AIDS is a man-made disease. To this day I remain convinced the theory is the most logical one for this unprecedented disease that has killed millions around the world. In 1988, my book *AIDS and the Doctors of Death* was published, followed by *Queer Blood* in 1993. My research on this subject continues to this day, and all of it is available for study on various web sites on the Internet.

In the 1970s, the decade before AIDS, virologists were busy trying to determine if human cancer was caused by viruses similar to certain tumors that were caused by known animal cancer viruses. In this research human cancer tissue and blood was transferred into various species of animals. Animal cancer-causing viruses were adapted to human cells in cell culture, and animal viruses from different species were mixed together, forming new "hybrid" and "recombinant" viruses.

Virologists also realized that seemingly normal cells could contain genetic information placed within them by a virus many cell generations before. As a result, much research centered around looking for pieces of viral genetic information in normal and in malignant cells. Animal cancer viruses like the Rous sarcoma virus and others were used as agents to change or alter the genes of cells.

Genetic engineering was inherently dangerous because deadly agents were combined which could have serious consequences if they escaped from these virus laboratories into the environment. These new viral creations were also of great interest to the biological warfare scientists, particularly after 1971 when the Army's biowarfare research unit at Ft. Detrick, Maryland, was combined with cancer research at the National Cancer Institute.

Because the cancer microbe is unrecognized in the scientific community, there has obviously been no concern about passing these pleomorphic bacteria and their "virus-sized" components into new species of animals through the process of "species jumping"—via human and animal viral laboratory experimentation. Livingston and Alexander-Jackson believed that the "virus particles" observed by virologists in cancer were, in reality, the "virus-like" forms of *P. cryptocides.*

In a recently published book, *AIDS: What the Discoverers of HIV Never Admitted; Is AIDS Really Caused by a Virus?,* author Lawrence Broxmeyer, M.D., actually proclaims that the cause of AIDS is Livingston's cancer microbe, as evidenced by the acid-fast bacteria I discovered in AIDS-damaged tissue. He hypothesizes that AIDS is actually caused by immune-suppressing atypical acid-fast mycobacteria, particularly *Mycobacterium avium*. Broxmeyer believes HIV merely represents a virus particle derived from the tiniest filterable forms of acid-fast bacteria. He thinks that Gallo and Montagnier discovered a virus because that was the only thing they were looking for.

Livingston would undoubtedly agree that HIV is the virus-like form of *Progenitor cryptocides*, and I would speculate that such a "new" sexually-transmissible form of *P. cryptocides* could have been engineered in a virus laboratory and introduced into select human populations, as scientists have done surreptitiously for decades.

The End of Cancer Microbe Research

Virginia wrote in *The Conquest of Cancer* that "I am confident that all my findings will be universally corroborated and that my treatment methods, or close variations thereof, will eventually become the prevalent treatment of cancer." She was concerned about environmental issues and ensuing future health problems of people, but more importantly, she asked: "But what are we to do *now*?"

After four decades of cancer microbe research, she proposed all infants be immunized at birth with vaccines specifically developed against *P. cryptocides*. We should also eliminate cancer from our food chain by vaccinating cattle and chickens, and feed our food animals with uncontaminated materials. [This was years before Mad Cow Disease.] We should immunize our pets to stop cross-infection. We should control the chemicalization of our fruit trees, plants and vegetables by promoting the use of natural deterrents. We should promote, not criticize, diets that are vegetarian or composed mostly of natural foods and raw vegetables. We should assume greater control of toxic materials used by industry and control the petro-chemicals in our environment.

In her last few years, Virginia was surrounded by lawyers making deals to patent her animal vaccines that were apparently successful in decreasing the incidence of animal cancer. The legal team advised her not to talk publicly about her current vaccine activities. It seemed that all the scientists were now patenting their discoveries to protect their research and to make more money. So much of science was now "secret" due to proprietary concerns. In the high-tech and bio-tech world of the 1980s, medical science and medical practice had become big business, more interested in profits than patients. Virginia's vaccine to prevent Marek's disease (a cancerous disease in poultry) was licensed in 1986, and she was hopeful about patenting another vaccine for cows.

I gathered she was making lots of money. The Wheelers now drove a Rolls Royce, the only time in my life that I have ridden in one. They were building a huge new home in exclusive Rancho Santa Fe. Business was booming at the clinic with several new physicians hired to help with the patient load. She was ecstatic about the success of her many real estate investments, and about the shopping center she just bought.

But the professional animosity against her treatment methods continued with a vengeance. That same year, the government actively began investigating her clinic, determined to put a stop to the vaccines she was using. The medical establishment cannot successfully attack renegade physicians for their ideas, but when doctors utilize unproven and untested therapies, the medical authorities can make things extremely unpleasant.

Virginia's vaccines were made from *Progenitor* bacteria cultured from the patient's own body fluids, usually from urine. After the bacteria were cultured, they were killed by heating or formaldehyde, and then diluted and injected back into the patient—with the hope that it would stimulate the immune system to produce an antibody response against the cancer bacteria. Virginia stressed that the vaccine was used to stimulate the immune system, but the vaccine became widely regarded as an "anti-cancer vaccine" by her enemies.

I believe the vaccine idea originally came from Eleanor, although I know Seibert also believed vaccines could be highly successful in treating cancer. The "autogenous" and killed-bacterial vaccines were first successfully introduced and administered by Dr. W. M. Crofton of Edinburgh, Scotland. Virginia and Eleanor believed that a vaccine, "tailor made" to the patient's own specific microbes, could be an efficient immunizing agent against cancer and related diseases.

For 15 years Virginia used autogenous vaccines at the Livingston Clinic. Although the efficacy of the vaccine was unproven, it certainly was not harmful because it was made from the patient's own bacteria. Nevertheless, the cancer establishment felt threatened by Virginia's use of untested vaccines year after year in her practice. No doubt some physicians were also angered by her success with some patients, and jealous of her financial success.

For decades the government had spent billions of dollars supporting cancer research, but not a dime was ever spent researching the microbiology of cancer. At her own expense, Virginia was expected to prove to the National Cancer Institute and finally to the Food and Drug Administration that her vaccines were safe and effective. Such proof of a vaccine's safety and efficacy could take years and was hugely expensive.

In a front page news story titled "Skeptical scientists test alleged 'cancer vaccine'" (San Diego *Union Tribune*, November 28, 1986), former chairman of the California Advisory Council, Dr. Wallace Simpson, claimed, "I think what she's doing is unscientific and quackery." In defense Livingston confessed to the reporter, "For a long time I didn't want to come out openly and fight anyone, but now I think I have to. I can't take that, being called fraudulent." A photo of Virginia showed a white-haired and white lab-coated, dejected old woman leaning against a wall. The caption read: "Livingston-Wheeler, Genius or Quack?"

In 1987 there was a court hearing in San Francisco to review her clinic activities. Virginia asked if I would testify. I flew to the bay city and told the judge that I greatly respected Dr. Livingston and held her cancer research in the highest regard. He seemed sympathetic. I am sure it must have been a very expensive court case to fight, and very stressful.

I am sure Virginia was bitter in her final years, as she had every right to be. She had devoted more than 40 years to researching the microbe that causes cancer. At the end she was rejected by her colleagues as a quack and a fraud, and hounded by the government as a perceived criminal.

In 1987, Owen Wheeler's malignant lymphoma returned and he died of complications in December, at the age of 79. Irene Diller passed away in 1988 at age 88. At age 81, Virginia was devastated. The following year she married for the fifth time, to a man thirty years younger. I met him twice, and I couldn't imagine them having much in common. But Virginia craved male companionship and she seemed content being with him. I was told he was the pool man she employed at her newly built home in Rancho Santa Fe, north of San Diego.

Ralph M. Moss, author of *The Cancer Industry* (1980), a highly unflattering report of the cancer establishment, hosts a website. According to Moss, in February 1990, California Health Director Kenneth W. Kizer issued an order requiring the Livingston Clinic to "cease and desist from prescribing and using autogenous vaccines in treating patients." Livingston was never contacted by the authorities before the order was implemented. Nor were there any patient complaints about the clinic or its treatment. This prosecution by the California health department was a nightmare for Virginia.

In March, Dr. Virginia made the trek to Washington and spoke eloquently at the Office of Technology Assessment hearing and received an ovation for her defiant speech. When at her best, she could still demonstrate great warmth and spontaneity. The following month the author received a late night telephone call from Virginia congratulating him on the revised, paperback edition of *The Cancer Industry*. Ralph Moss was a great fan of her work and wrote a highly flattering portrait of her in his book. He fondly remembers Virginia as a great person and a great scientist, who sadly never received the recognition she deserved in her lifetime. He predicts the true scope of her achievements will only become known in years to come.

Virginia got in serious trouble with the government for her autogenous vaccines, but she never caused deaths with her vaccines. The following year Robert Gallo and the National Institutes of Health were severely criticized for several deaths caused by an experimental and unapproved AIDS vaccine. In a July 7, 1991, report in the *Chicago Tribune* titled "U.S. Agency Faulted in AIDS Vaccine Study," John Crewdson reported that the NIH did not adequately protect human subjects during these experiments. An NIH oversight committee ordered NIH director Bernadine Healy to develop, within two months, a comprehensive plan for bringing all human experimentation by NIH researchers into accord with federal regulations. "Dr. Robert C. Gallo and Dr. Daniel Zagury of the University of Paris, are the two scientists the panel singled out for criticism in its 21-page report. The report criticizes Zagury for several violations, including failing to inform American authorities of the deaths of three French volunteers on whom Zagury tested an experimental AIDS vaccine developed with Gallo. Three months prior to learning of the Paris deaths, NIH stopped all research collaborations between Gallo and Zagury after finding several violations of federal and research regulations in the United States and France."

In early 1990 my book, *The Cancer Microbe*, was published. It included biographical sketches of Livingston, Alexander-Jackson, Diller and Seibert, and other medical greats who studied the hidden killer in cancer.

On May 22, 1990, Eleanor Alexander-Jackson passed away in Saskatoon, Canada. Her son Togwell wrote me how pleased he was that I devoted space for her in my book. "It is encouraging to learn that Mother's work is being recognized and appreciated by a younger generation of doctors. It would be very gratifying to see all the pioneers of the germ theory of cancer—my mother, Dr. Livingston, Dr.Crofton, and the rest—finally receive their rightful place in medical history."

On a trip abroad with daughter Julie Wagner, Virginia suffered a massive coronary and died on June 30, 1990, in Athens. Her life was marked by the greatest scientific discovery of the century. But there was no recognition of this tremendous achievement, only rejection from the profession of medicine that she dearly loved. Ironically, her life ended at age 83 in Greece—the land of the world's best-known human tragedies.

Also in 1990, at the age of 92, Florence Seibert was inducted into the National Women's Hall of Fame, along with Barbara Jordan (government), Billie Jean King (athletics) and Margaret Bourke-White (arts). When she passed away in 1991, her death was noted in *Time* and *People* magazines, and in major newspapers, such as the *Los Angeles Times*. All the obituaries mentioned her contributions to the safety of intravenous fluids and her great achievement with the tuberculosis skin test. But not a word was written about her cancer microbe research, to which she devoted the last 30 years of her life.

Within a period of three years, Irene Diller, Eleanor Alexander-Jackson, Virginia Livingston and Florence Seibert were all gone. The Golden Age of the microbiology of cancer had passed without notice.

In 1994, after 29 years as a dermatologist at Kaiser-Permanente, I retired. In 2003 my partner was diagnosed with prostate cancer. He opted for surgical removal of the prostate. Fortunately, there was no evidence of spread of the cancer outside of the prostate gland. I respectfully asked the pathologist to order a special acid-fast Fite stain of the prostate gland, so that I could study it for bacteria. Placing a drop of oil on the prepared slides, I carefully studied Frank's gland containing the cancer tumor. Within a few minutes I found round intra-cellular and extra-cellular, variably sized coccoid forms so typical of the cancer germs that I had discovered in many different kinds of cancer. Privately, I contacted microscopist James Solliday to photograph the microbes. Jim took some splendid digital color microphotographs and presented them to me on a computer compact disc. Now I had the ability to send photos of cancer microbes via computer to anyone in the world. Quite a change from my first studies in the 1960s, when such things were impossible.

I thought the finding of microbes in prostate cancer might interest a few physicians. After all, almost every man, if he lives long enough, will develop prostate cancer and so many men's lives (and their sex lives) are ruined by the current brutal treatment of prostate cancer. According to the American Cancer Society, in 2002 there were 220,000 diagnosed cases of prostate cancer in the U.S., and 29,000 deaths.

I showed the photographs to several urologists and emailed photos to a number of physicians and researchers on the Internet that had special interest in prostate cancer. None of the urologists showed any great interest, but they admitted they had never seen anything like the tiny forms I showed them in the acid-fast stained tissue sections. They said they had never studied prostate cancer with an acid-fast stain. None of the physicians on the net responded to my emails.

After four decades of research I was not terribly surprised by the disinterest of my colleagues. Doctors hate to be challenged, and they will quickly turn off to controversial ideas, and the subject of "cancer microbes" is strictly taboo in medical science.

I once bluntly asked a pathologist if she had seen the

acid-fast forms that I was observing in all kinds of cancer, and she finally admitted that she did. I then asked why she did not include these forms in any of her reports. She said she was not sure what they represented and they were not something known to pathologists. She was supportive of my research, however, and said perhaps one day I would win a Nobel Prize for my discoveries. I wasn't sure if she was serious or joking, but I knew the conversation was over and to continue to press the issue would be futile and argumentative.

In areas of science that are controversial, you simply cannot push physicians. But it is always sad for me when physicians totally ignore bacteria in cancer. That's one of the reasons why I have few close friends who are doctors. Most are so terribly closed-minded, and it is rare to encounter a physician who thinks differently from the herd. It is even more rare for such a physician to speak out. I can certainly understand the reasons for this, but I think this is why the cause of diseases like cancer is so poorly understood, and why the treatment of cancer is still so barbaric.

Without the powerful presence and energy of Dr. Virginia, the clinic on Duke Street was never quite the same. It continued to operate until 2004, when it closed its doors forever.

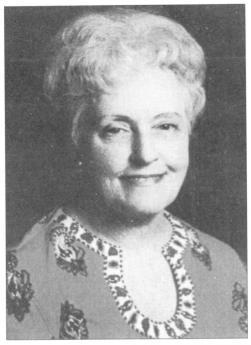

Virginia Livingston, M.D., (1906-1990)
undated photo, circa 1965.

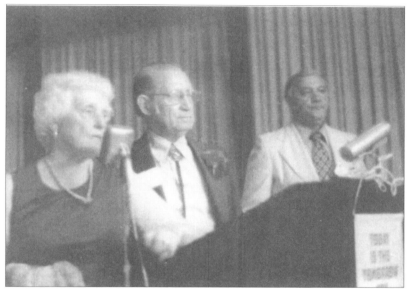

Virginia Livingston and her husband Owen Wheeler, M.D. and John Steinbacher, at a Cancer Federation Conference in 1980.

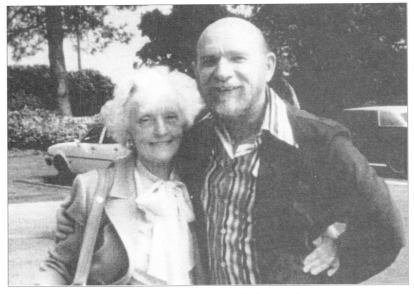

Virginia Livingston and the author.
San Diego, March 1981.

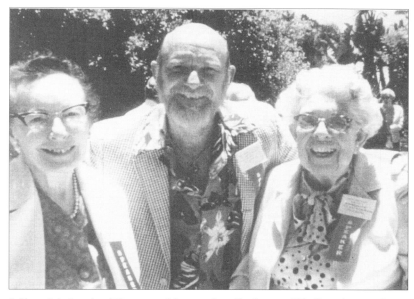

Microbiologist Eleanor Alexander-Jackson, Ph.D., the author,
and cytologist Irene Corey Diller, Ph.D., at an International
Symposium on the Diagnosis and Treatment of Cancer and
Allied Diseases, sponsored by the Livingston-Wheeler
Foundation, San Diego, CA, June 1980.

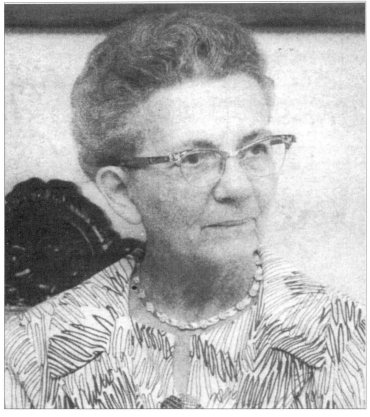

Florence B. Seibert, Ph.D., Biochemist, (1897-1991). Seibert
developed the first accurate skin test for tuberculosis, which is
still used around the world. In August, 1990, at the age of 92,
she was inducted into the The National Woman's Hall of Fame,
in Seneca Falls, New York, along with Barbara Jordan
(Government), Billie Jean King (Athletics) and
Margaret Bourke-White (Arts).

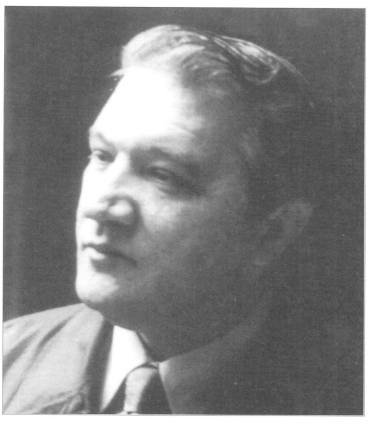

John Steinbacher, founder of the Cancer Federation, Inc. in 1977 in Banning, California. The Federation began as a charitable organization highly supportive of research in the field of cancer immunology, and sympathetic to Livingston's view of the infectious origin of cancer.

CHAPTER THREE

Bacteria, Cancer, and the Origin of Life

The cancer microbe studied for more than a century is undoubtedly the most important microbe in man, even though it remains totally unrecognized and unappreciated by medical science. To Livingston and Jackson, *Progenitor cryptocides* was the germ that allowed life to reproduce itself, but in old age it was also the taker of life. Modern day virologists probing with the tiniest of viral forms are unlocking mysteries of heredity, cancer and life itself. But the two women considered so-called cancer viruses as representing the tiniest elements of the Pc microbe.

Years ago, on a rainy afternoon in Virginia's library, we were alone together, musing about cancer microbe research and the hostility of physicians regarding cancer-causing bacteria. In the quiet time between us, we began to ponder the meaning of life. What was it all about? It was all as mysterious to her as it is to the rest of us.

Is new life merely just the beginning of eventual death, as scientists believe? Or is death the beginning of "eternal life," as some religions teach? Could life be a never-ending cycle of life/death/life/death reincarnations? Can life develop from non-living things, or was all life and the universe created eons ago by the Creator, or through some freak accident of the cosmos? Where do I come from? What will happen to me after death? These are unsolvable questions human beings have asked themselves for centuries.

I wonder what Virginia's place will be in medical history. With so many new, remarkable discoveries taking place in bacteriology, I can't help but think that her ideas will fit perfectly into the science of the future.

Nanobacteria, NASA and Astrobiology

Robert Folk is a geologist who specializes in microscopic examinations of limestones. Working in Italy in the 1980s with a new scanning electron microscope (SEM) with magnifications up to 100,000X, he repeatedly came across "hordes of tiny bumps and balls" entombed within the rock. Initially he passed it off as artifacts or laboratory contamination, as had every other geologist using the SEM. However, after a year of doubts and some reading in microbiology, Folk learned that exceedingly small cells called "ultramicrobacteria" did in fact exist. With further microscopic work, he realized that the enormous numbers of tiny grape-like and chain-like clusters were indeed bacteria. Remarkably, these "nanobacteria" could be easily cultured as common forms of bacteria, known as cocci, bacilli, staphylococci and streptococci. Folk's first scientific presentation of these astounding findings was met with "stony silence" and "howls of disbelief" from microbiologists. To this day, some scientists contend so-called nanobacteria are simply too small to contain the necessary genetic material for life.

In microbiology, the ultramicroscopic bacteria are regarded as stressed or resting forms of big bacteria, and are thought to be both rare and dormant. Geologists prefer the spelling "nannobacteria" to conform with the spelling of extremely tiny "nannofossils," a common term in geology dating back to the nineteenth century. Folk claims nanobacteria are enormously abundant in minerals and rocks, and that they form most of the world's bio-mass. If so, how could they have been missed for so long? Folk says microbiologists have little or no interest in bacteria found in soils or rocks; and for fifty years it has been standard microbiological dogma that bacteria smaller than 0.2 micrometers cannot exist.

Size does matter, even when discussing the tiniest forms of life. The term "ultramicroscopic" is applied to bacterial cells smaller than 0.3 micrometers. At this size, bacteria are still barely visible as the tiniest of dots discernable with the light microscope. The ordinary light microscope can magnify objects up to 1000X, but objects smaller than 0.25 micrometers cannot be seen. The electron microscope is able to photograph objects at magnifications of 300,000X, or higher.

Nanobacteria are the smallest of living creatures, measuring in the 0.05 to 0.2 micrometer range. (A micrometer is 1/1000 of a millimeter). This puts nanobacteria as an intermediate life-form between normal bacteria and viruses. Viruses are around 0.01 to 0.02 micrometers in size and cannot be seen with the ordinary light optical microscope.

The size of bacteria, nanobacteria, and viruses, is exceedingly important to bear in mind because the "dividing line" between bacteriology and virology has been the customary "filter pore size" of 0.2 micrometers. Microbiologists have always assumed that such a filter pore will catch all bacteria, and that a fluid running through a 0.2 micrometer filter pore would be bacteria-free. Therefore, when geologists photographed 0.1 micrometer "bumps" they simply passed them off as contamination, never believing that they could be living bacteria. Folk says, "You see what you are looking for and what you have faith in!"

By the early 1990s these nanobacteria were investigated by a team of biologists in Finland, headed by Olavi Kajander. Nanobacteria have now been found in kidney stones, dental plaque, the gall bladder, in calcified arteries and heart valves, and in certain skin diseases. Kajander's team also reported nanobacterial forms as small as 0.05 microns in human blood.

Most disturbing are reports showing nanobacterial contamination of fetal bovine serum used in the production of many viral vaccines. This adds concern to the controversial problem of "vaccine-induced illness" and the fear that some people have of contaminated vaccines. Are nanobacteria connected with the origin of life on Earth? Nanobacteria-like "fossils" have been observed in several meteors, such as the Martian meteorite found on the Antarctic ice shelf in 1984. This meteorite is believed to be 4.5 billion years old, and is thought to have left Mars 16 million years ago. Supporters of nanobacteria research insist these bacteria have implications for how life began on Earth, and on planets like Mars.

NASA, the U.S. space agency, has an Astrobiology Roadmap program, which consists of more than 200 scientists and technologists. Astrobiology addresses three basic questions: How does life begin and evolve? Does life exist elsewhere in the universe? What is the future of life on Earth and beyond?

According to Roadmap, there are revolutionary changes going on in microbiology. "Our ongoing exploration has led to continued discoveries of life in environments that have been previously considered uninhabitable. For example, we find thriving communities (of microbes) in the boiling hot springs of Yellowstone, the frozen deserts of Antarctica, the concentrated sulfuric acid in acid-mine drainages, and the ionizing radiation fields in nuclear reactors. We find some microbes that grow in the deepest parts of the ocean and require 500 to 1,000 bars of hydrostatic pressure. Life has evolved strategies that allow it to survive even beyond the daunting physical and chemical limits to which it has adapted to grow. To survive, organisms can assume forms that enable them to withstand freezing, complete desiccation, starvation, high levels of radiation exposure, and other physical and chemical challenges."

In addition, astrobiologists tell us that huge amounts of bacteria and possibly viruses are contained in Earth's upper atmosphere. It is estimated that a ton of these organisms arrive on Earth every day!

Communication between Bacteria

In an amazing discovery, scientists have learned that bacteria can communicate with each another. When enough microbes gather to form a "quorum," they release a hormone (a pheromone) which allows them to "talk" to one another and plan strategies, and even make some genetic changes to allow survival. Not only do similar bacteria talk to each other, they also talk between species. Barbara Bassler, a molecular biologist at Princeton, is a leading pioneer in quorum sensing. Writing about her work for *Wired* magazine (April 2003), Steve Silberman says that communicating microbes are able to collectively track changes in their environment, conspire with other species, build mutually beneficial alliances with other types of bacteria, gain advantages over competitors, and communicate with their hosts—the sort of collective strategizing typically ascribed to bees, ants, and people, not to bacteria." Quorum sensing has profound implications in the war against disease, particularly now that so many bacteria are becoming resistant to antibiotics. Not everyone in microbiology is convinced that bacteria can communicate. But why can't bacterial cells talk to one another? Don't all the cells in our body "talk" to each other in some way?

Viruses, Bacteria, and the Beginnings of Life

Charles Darwin's *Origin of the Species* was published in 1859 and is the seminal book that gave rise to biology, as well as to the scientific and religious controversies that continue to this day. People were incensed to think humans could have arisen from monkeys and apes. Now some scientists think we developed side-by-side along with bacteria.

Every human, plant and animal cell has genetic material inside a nucleus. Surrounding the nucleus is a jelly-like cytoplasm which contains the "mitochondria," which are considered to be tiny chemical factories that process the nutrients that provide energy to the cell.

Evolutionary biologist Lynn Margulis of the University of Massachusetts believes the ancestors of all life are the bacteria, which fused into higher forms of life. Margulis follows in the footsteps of American biologist Ivan Wallin, who in 1927 first claimed that mitochondria originated as free-living bacteria. Wallin thought that ancient bacteria and their host cells evolved together to establish an inseparable symbiotic partnership. He even claimed to have removed mitochondria from cells and to grow them. Needless to say, Wallin's ideas were ridiculed and almost universally rejected.

But Margulis also theorizes that the origin of the mitochondria in our cells is derived from separate organisms that long-ago moved into other cells and entered a symbiotic (sort of a co-dependant) relationship with multi-cellular forms of life. Remarkably, the DNA in the mitochondria is totally different than the DNA in the rest of the cell, which lends support to this idea.

Margulis subscribes to the vision that the Earth, as a whole, is a living being. In *What Is Life?* (1955), co-written with Dorion Sagan, she maintains that all life is bacteria— or descends from bacteria. In short, life *is* bacteria. And, as such, bacteria are closer to immortality than animals with bodies.

Bacteria account for the vast majority of life forms on Earth, and are essential to maintain the conditions for life on the planet. They are the smallest living cells that can replicate without a nucleus, and are indeed the building-blocks of life.

What can microbes tell us about our origin and our destinies? Could we be immortal like our one-celled ancestors?

Creating "Life" in the Laboratory

What is the lowest form of life? Can life be created from non-life? Some scientists believe viruses are the lowest form of life. We are told viruses need to penetrate a cell and use the cell's genes to survive. In the process, disease can be produced. But are viruses "alive" or "dead"? Scientists can't agree on this.

In 1991 Eckard Wimmer and his associates created a

polio virus for the very first time—outside a cell and in a test tube. They extracted a soup of proteins from human cells, and then added genetic material from a polio virus. After a few hours, fully assembled polio viruses appeared in the mix.

According to a *New York Times* report (Dec. 13, 1991), Wimmer was asked, "Is the product in the test tube living or nonliving?" Some consider viruses to be simple living organisms, others consider viruses to be very complicated chemicals, said Wimmer. But "when it hits the cell it is very much alive. Some argue that one attribute of life is that it can reproduce itself. Well, that is what viruses do when they get into the cells. The debate on whether viruses are alive has been going on since they were discovered 100 years ago."

Although the cause of most cancers remains a mystery, research over the past half-century has focused on cancer viruses as a probable cause. With research focused on viruses, it would seem ludicrous to ask, "Can bacteria cause cancer?"

The mere thought of bacteria causing cancer drives most cancer experts up the wall! However, with the recent interest in nanobacteria and their discovery in the blood and in various diseases of unknown origin, the question should not be so easily dismissed. Furthermore, in the past decade physicians have come to accept the fact that stomach ulcers can be produced by bacteria (*Helicobacter pylori*), and some ulcers eventually lead to stomach cancer. For many decades it was dogma that bacteria could not live in the acid environment of the stomach. Furthermore, pathologists could never see or detect bacteria in the stomach lining around ulcers. With the discovery of Helicobacteria and special staining techniques, doctors can now demonstrate bacteria in many ulcers—proving that microbiologists and pathologists were universally unable to "see" microbes, even though they existed in the ulcers. This is undoubtedly the case with cancer bacteria and the refusal or inability of scientists to "see" them, even though they are present in cancer.

Dogma and Heresies in Microbiology

After a century of "modern" medical science, we still don't know the cause of cancer, heart disease, and many other chronic diseases that kill millions of people every year. The reason for this, in my view, is that medical science refuses to recognize the role that microbes (smaller than bacteria and larger than viruses) play in these diseases. Much of the fault lies in the dogma left over from the nineteenth century by such scientific icons as Louis Pasteur and Robert Koch, who are revered as fathers of microbiology and bacteriology. At a time when viruses and nanobacteria and astrobiology were unknown and when "the germ theory of disease" was in its infancy, both scientists held rigid views as to what was possible and not possible in biology. Neither Pasteur nor Koch could fathom the concept that living organisms might arise from non-living sources.

Unfortunately, Pasteur (1822-1895), despite all his achievements, was not a medical doctor (as many people erroneously believe) and had no medical training. He was consumed with fermentation experiments and with proving "air germs" were the basis for human disease, although he provided no explanation for the origin of atmospheric germs or how life began on Earth. Koch (1843-1910), who discovered the bacteria that caused tuberculosis, was obsessed with classifying microbes grown in the laboratory into exact species, depending on their size, structure, physical, and chemical properties. He insisted the species that were created were pure and stable; and that species were unable to change back and forth between each other. According to Koch, each species of bacteria produced a separate and distinct disease. Each germ also had to originate from similar "parent" germs—which reproduced by dividing in half by "binary fission."

Not every physician of that era believed all the pronouncements of Pasteur and Koch. A few physician-scientists challenged them because they knew what was often "proven" in laboratory experiments might not always be applicable to what was going on with bacteria hidden within the human body.

Antoine Bechamp (1816-1908), no slouch in the science department, was well known as a scientific rival of the famous Pasteur. The Frenchman was not only a Doctor of Medicine and Science, but at various times was also Professor of Medical Chemistry and Pharmacology, and Professor of Physics, Toxicology, and Biological Chemistry. There is also some evidence that Pasteur plagiarized much of Bechamp's original research.

Pasteur, however, is credited in history with saving the French beer, wine and silkworm industries, and with pasteurization and vaccine research. Bechamp, despite his brilliance, was eventually eclipsed by the younger man. The details of the scientific controversy and plagiarism accusations are chronicled in E. Douglas Hume's book, *Bechamp or Pasteur? A Lost Chapter in the History of Biology* (1923), remarkably still in print.

Bechamp had his own ideas concerning the origin of life and the germ theory of disease. In animal and plant cells he observed infinitesimal microscopic "granulations" that he considered the incorruptible elements of all life. After many laboratory experiments and microscopic examinations of these granules, the physician-scientist claimed these so-called "microzymas" were capable of developing into common living organisms that go by the name of bacteria.

In Bechamp's view, Pasteur's "air germs" had nothing to do with the origin and appearance of these microzymas in tissue. In fact, Bechamp wrote that Pasteur's air germs most likely derived from dying life-forms. Like Folk a century later, Bechamp found barely visible microzymas/ bacteria in chalk and limestone that he interpreted as survivor life-forms of past ages. Although all the microzymas looked similar, they varied in their chemical abilities. Each tissue, or organ, or gland had microzymas that differed from each other.

Hume claims Bechamp and his colleagues showed these tiny microzymas were, in reality, "organised ferments" with the potential to develop into bacteria. In this development, they passed through certain inter-mediary stages. Some of these intermediate bacterial stages were regarded by people like Koch as different species, but to Bechamp they were all related and derived from microzymas. Adding more heresy to Pasteur's dogma, Bechamp wrote that without oxygen, microzymas do not die; they go into a state of rest. Bechamp preached, "Every living being has arisen from the microzymas, and every living being is reducible to the microzymas."

Like Bechamp, Henry Charlton Bastian's (1837-1915) studies investigating the origin of life were closely tied into his understanding of the origin of infectious disease. He was also the last of the great scientists to uphold the theory of "spontaneous regeneration," by concluding that life could come from non-life. Bastian argued that microorganisms were produced as by-products of the disease process, not as opportunistic infections, but from degenerating tissue by a process termed "heterogenesis." Heterogenesis is the idea that living organisms can arise without parents from organic starting materials—an idea certainly not in accord with Pasteur and Koch.

Bechamp and Bastian's research was also a threat to the followers of Charles Darwin (1809-1882), whose evolutional theories revolutionized science. Like Pasteur, Darwin was not a medical doctor and had no training in human pathology. *And* while doctors like Bechamp and Bastian and others were discovering new forms of life emanating from human diseased tissue and from the bowels of limestone, Pasteur, Koch and the Darwinians simply disregarded all this in favor of their own research and pronouncements.

Bastian paid dearly for his unorthodoxy (and for some well publicized but failed experiments), and his once-famous name is largely forgotten. Microbiologist and science professor James Strick has recently revived interest in Bastian's books on the origin of life, and a six-volume set reprinting much of his work has been recently published. Strick is also the author of *Sparks of Life* (2000), which chronicles the famous nineteenth century scientific and bacteriologic debates over Darwinism and spon-taneous generation.

Pleomorphism and the Classification of Bacteria

Koch, famous for his tuberculosis discoveries, was rigid in his belief that a specific germ had only one form (monomorphism). He opposed all research showing that some germs had more than one form (pleomorphism) and complex "life cycles." Thus, from the very beginning of bacteriology there was conflict between the monomorphists and the pleomorphists, with the former totally overruling the latter and dominating microbiology to this day.

In the attempt to "classify" bacteria as the lowest forms of life known at that time, there was no consideration given to any possible connection between the various species of bacteria. The dogma was that a coccus remained a coccus, a rod remained a rod, and there was no interplay between them. There was no "crossing" from one species to another, and the research of the pleomorphists that suggested otherwise was ignored.

When viruses were discovered they were made separate from bacteria, although bacteria are also known to be susceptible to viral infection. Viruses were put in one box; bacteria in another. As a result, the spectacular number of "filterable" pleomorphic microbial forms that form a bridge between the "living" bacteria and the "dead" viruses are still largely unstudied and considered of no great importance in clinical medicine.

When culturing specimens from patients, most doctors simply want to know the name of the microbe cultured in the lab and what antibiotics the germ is "sensitive" to. Thanks to Pasteur, common "skin" bacteria like cocci and bacilli are often viewed as suspicious "contaminants" or "secondary invaders" or "opportunistic infections" of no great importance as etiologic agents.

"Koch's postulates" became the required laboratory procedure to prove that a specific microbe causes a specific disease, but the postulates did not work very well for viruses. Even when filterable pleomorphic bacteria were shown to cause disease and Koch's postulates were fulfilled, the research was still generally ignored because such germs were not considered "valid" life-forms.

As a result of all this dogma and rigidity, medical thought was completely turned off to the possibility that cancer was caused by bacteria. But to the minds of some medical heretics, these century-old scientific beliefs were wrong, wrong, wrong!

Cancer, New Life, and Reich's "T-Bacilli"

Although the origin and cause of cancer is mysterious, there is no doubt that cancer is the body's futile and often fatal attempt to create new life and new growth. *That is why cancer is so intimately connected with theories about the origin of life.*

One of the most controversial physicians of the last century was Wilhelm Reich (1897-1957), a psychiatrist and cancer researcher who claimed to discover "orgone energy"—an energy that pervades the world and is intimately connected with our physical and mental well being. In *The Cancer Biopathy* (1948), he wrote that cancer is a systemic disease caused by emotional despair and resignation and the chronic thwarting of natural sexual functioning. These were just a few of his highly unorthodox beliefs based on his many observations and experiments.

Reich also uncovered infectious "T-bacilli" (bacteria) in cancer that resulted from the degeneration of cancerous tissue. In his view, these bacteria formed a bridge between the living and the non-living. The T-bacilli were present in the blood and tissue *before* the cancer tumor developed, and these microbes were intimately connected to "bions" and the loss of biological energy. Reich's heretical bions were the carriers of biological energy; and the staphylococcus and streptococcus germs that he found connected to cancer were actually formed from the degeneration of the bions.

Just as there is no clear dividing line between life and non-life, there is no clear boundary between healthy and diseased individuals. Reich claimed the cancer cell developed as the body's attempt to resist the build-up of the T-bacilli in energy-depleted tissue. "The first step in the development of the cancer tumor is not the cancer cell…it is the appearance of T-bacilli in the tissue or in the blood." But T-bacilli were not only found in cancer; they were also present in the blood and tissues of both healthy and sick non-cancerous individuals. However, sick and cancerous patients showed a larger number of these forms, and Reich developed a blood test to show this. T-bacilli were always found where there is degeneration of protein, and in that respect, Reich wrote, "All humans have cancer."

The orgone energy of the body determined the resistance of the body to these microbes. As long as the tissues and blood are "organotically strong, every T-bacillus will be destroyed and eliminated before it can propagate, accumulate, and cause damage," wrote Reich. Because cancer germs were present in healthy people, Reich knew this would be a very difficult concept for physicians to consider and accept.

Reich wanted scientists to look at science in a new way and to try and see it from the point of view of "energetic functionalism." For example, "The bacteriologist sees the staphylococcus as a static formation, spherical or oval in shape, about 0.8 micron in size, reacting with a bluish coloration to Gram stain, and arranged in clusters. These characteristics are important for orgone biophysics, but are not the essentials. The name itself says nothing about the origin, function, and position of the blue coccus in nature. What the bacteriologists calls 'staphylococcus' is, for orgone physics, a small energy vesicle in the process of degeneration. Orgone biophysics investigates the origin of the staphylococcus from other forms of life and follows its transformation. It examines the staphylococcus in connection with the processes of the total biological energy of the organism and produces it experimentally through degenerative processes in bions, cells, etc." Through his scientific experiments with orgone energy, Reich hoped to harness orgone for the treatment of disease and the good of humanity.

Needless to say, Reich's entire life's work was considered hogwash, and a scientific inquisition eventually ensued. Branded a menace and a quack, he ran afoul of the Food and Drug Administration (FDA) which claimed his experimental "orgone accumulator" was being used illegally to treat cancer—and that it was nothing more than a perverted sex box. Refusing to obey a court injunction, Reich was tried and sentenced to prison. His books were burned and his equipment destroyed by FDA agents. He died at the federal penitentiary at Lewisburg, Pennsylvania, in March 1957, at age 60.

His research into the origin of life, and his belief that the orgone energy contained within the tiniest forms of life could not be destroyed, make him one of the most misunderstood and hated physicians of the twentieth century.

It is interesting to note that Virginia and Eleanor and Reich all resided in the New York City area during the late 1940s and early 1950s. One wonders what might have resulted if all three controversial researchers had collaborated on the cancer problem.

Cancer and the Cancer Microbe

As some scientists are finally realizing, there is a large realm of microbial life-forms that lies between "bacteria" and "viruses." Within this relatively uncharted never-never land of microbiology lies the biologic secrets of life, disease, cancer, death, regeneration, and perhaps even immortality itself.

Livingston and Jackson were among the first to suggest that certain "cancer viruses," as well as certain cell-wall-deficient bacteria (mycoplasma), might all be related to a specific type of acid-fast bacteria isolated from various cancers.

Livingston believed everyone carried cancer microbes in their blood and tissues. In 1974, she discovered that cancer-associated bacteria produced an HCG-like hormone—the human choriogonadotropin hormone, which is an essential hormone needed to start life in the womb. She also thought the microbe was the germ that destroyed life as people aged. The microbe was Mother Nature's built-in terminator to force old people off the planet in order to make room for new life on the planet.

Even though Livingston's research was published for three decades in reputable medical journals, the American Cancer Society still claims her "cancer microbe" does not exist. An ACS-sponsored internet web page states: "One report on the bacteria *Progenitor cryptocides*, which Dr. Livingston-Wheeler claimed caused cancer, found that the bacteria does not exist but is actually a mixture of several different types of bacteria which Dr. Livingston-Wheeler labeled as one." The author of the ACS report is listed as "anonymous."

Over the past four decades I have tried to keep cancer microbe research alive by showing pleomorphic cancer bacteria in human cancer and in certain other diseases of unknown origin. In my research I have observed germs grown in the lab from cancerous tissue. Frequently they grow as simple round cocci, or as a mixture of cocci and rod-shaped bacilli, and rarely as streptococci. From diseases like scleroderma, I have seen "old" cultures evolve into peculiar and highly pleomorphic fungus-like "actinomycete" organisms, or evolve into bacteria resembling tuberculosis-type bacteria. Not infrequently, expert microbiologists could not agree on what to name these pleomorphic bacteria.

I have seen microbes change from one species to another, depending on what they are fed in the laboratory —staphylococcus germs that turn into rod-forms of corynebacteria—and revert back again to "pure" staphylococcus, depending on the lab media for growth. But most importantly, I have demonstrated these bacteria in acid-fast stained tissue sections of cancer, indicating that these microbes are not contaminants falling out of the air. Decade after decade of cancer microbe research remains forgotten, ignored, or overlooked because physicians cannot conceive of bacteria causing cancer.

Can Bacteria Cause Cancer? Alternative Medicine Confronts Big Science, was published by New York University Press in 1997. This investigation into the relationship between bacteria and chronic disease includes an excellent review of a century of cancer microbe research by anthropologist David J. Hess. As an advocate for alternative medicine, he maintains that economic and cultural values (rather than scientific values) have greatly influenced the rush towards radiation, chemotherapy, and toxic therapies as the only accepted treatment of cancer. Carefully examining the issue of bacterial vaccines and the connection between bacteria and chronic disease, Hess maintains that cancer microbe research has not only been dismissed, it has been actively suppressed by the cancer establishment.

Milton Wainwright, a microbiologist at the University of Sheffield, U.K., has written sympathetically about the bacteriology of cancer. Some of his recent publications include, "Nanobacteria and associated 'elementary bodies' in human disease and cancer" (1999), "The return of the cancer germ; Forgotten microbiology—back to the future" (2000), "Highly pleomorphic staphylococci as a cause of cancer" (2000), and "Is this the historical 'cancer germ'?" (2003).

Body Blood Bacteria

The idea that the blood contains bacteria related to cancer has been repeatedly raised by various cancer microbe researchers. However, the idea was never taken seriously because bacteria grown from cancer patients were never considered anything more than inconsequential contaminating bacteria, like staphylococci, streptococci, and various common bacilli presumed to be of no etiologic significance. Physicians still expect disease-causing bacteria to be of a specific species of bacterium which causes a "specific" disease. Physicians also believe each form of cancer is "different." Thus, the variety of different species of pleomorphic bacteria recovered from various cancers makes physicians highly dubious about a specific microbe causing a specific type of cancer.

In a series of papers (1970-1979) using the electron microscope and various testing procedures, an Italian team of researchers headed by Guido G. Tedeschi showed that the erythrocytes (red blood cells) and the blood platelets of both normal and diseased patients are cryptically infected with pleomorphic bacteria. Found within the erythrocytes were electron-dense "granular bodies," and a variety of microbial forms and species were reported as mycoplasma-like and corynebacteria-like L-forms (cell-wall-deficient forms) of bacteria, *Staphylococcus epidermidis*, micrococci, cocci, and cocco-bacillary forms. Such microbes are similar to what various cancer microbe researchers have reported over the past century. Some of Tedeschi's microbes were acid-fast, a staining quality characteristic of Livingston's cancer microbe.

All of this indicates that human blood is definitely not sterile, and should raise suspicion that these tiny blood bacteria could be involved in the production of disease— a conclusion Wilhelm Reich came to a half-century ago. Tedeschi's team suggested that the cocci and diphtheroid bacteria originated from cell-wall-deficient forms that were not related to a specific illness, but were the consequence of a "generalized crypto-infection."

A more recent study titled "Are there naturally occurring pleomorphic bacteria in the blood of healthy humans?" by R.W. McLaughlin and associates in the *Journal of Clinical Microbiology* (December 2002), confirms the presence of a wide diversity of micro-organisms within the blood of healthy people. With new research showing nanobacteria in the blood, it is apparent there is much to learn about the bacteriology of the blood and what microbes it contains normally, and what microbes it contains in disease.

As they have done for a century, microbiologists will undoubtedly continue quibbling about what to name these organisms. *But more important than a name is to determine what they do—not in the laboratory, but in the human body.* What is the energy force that allows these microbes to exist in harmony with us, and what turns them into killers?

Science, Soul, Spirit, and Immortality

Helena P. Blavatsky (1831-1891) is the controversial founder of the science of Theosophy, a philosophical and spiritual group with a keen interest in the origin of life. In researching Bastian on the Internet, I came across her name on a web page connected to his nineteenth century studies on tiny bacteria in limestone. Blavatsky's ideas about the origin of life are amazingly prophetic in light of current findings of nanobacteria in microbiology and geology. Her idea of a "vital force" also seems similar to Reich's "orgone energy."

Blavatsky wrote, "Life is not the expression of the organism, but, on the contrary, the organism is the expression of some prior and indestructible vital force. Nothing ever dies. Life's opposite is not death, but latency. Indeed, one is compelled to ask whether all humanity, past and future, is not imprisoned in latent form in the rocks and sands of our terrestrial sphere." In *The Secret Doctrine* (1888), she claims, "Everything that *is, was,* and *will be,* eternally IS, even the countless forms, which are finite and perishable only in their objective, not in their *ideal* Form. They existed as Ideas, in the Eternity, and, when they pass away, will exist as reflections."

Science has little or nothing to say about spirit, soul, and the hereafter. Skeptics are always seeking "proof." But if a disease like cancer is indeed caused by microscopic bacteria, it would indicate that physicians have been unable to see what was quite plain for some nineteenth and twentieth century scientists to observe using simple light microscopy. With powerful electron microscopes there is now little excuse for not "seeing" bacteria. With this in mind, it would behoove scientists, especially cancer experts, to do a little soul-searching (pun intentional).

In addition, scientists cannot seem to agree where life begins. So can we trust them completely to know when life ends? If human life continues after death, it must exist largely as energy. *And* can energy ever be destroyed? Einstein tells us that matter and energy are interconnected and are essentially different forms of the same thing. Physicists are excited about the possibilities of quantum physics, which is beyond my ken.

Professor of Mathematical Physics, Frank Tipler, confidently proclaims physics will lead to the immortality of humankind. In his controversial book *The Physics of Immortality* (1994) he states "Either theology is pure nonsense, a subject with no content, or else theology must ultimately become a branch of physics...The Goal of physics is understanding the ultimate nature of reality. If God is real, physicists will eventually find Him/Her."

After a lifetime meditating on the origin and meaning of life, I wondered if Virginia Livingston's scientific ideas had come the closest when she finally realized the cancer microbe was both the giver and the taker of life. And I remembered how Wilhelm Reich in his experiments could not destroy life and the orgone energy contained within it.

Although Virginia and I were 26 years apart there was an energy between us that seemed to spring from the same source. We were both born under the sign of Capricorn, and born to physician fathers who guided us into the noblest profession of healing. We both were easterners who went to medical school in New York City. She followed her father west in his later years, and my father followed me west in his later years. We both flourished professionally in Southern California in Los Angeles and San Diego. When I lived in San Diego for a year in 1959, she was living there. We both worked for Kaiser, she for a brief period, me for my entire career.

We both first discovered the cancer microbe by studying scleroderma, the rarest of skin diseases, and we each discovered the acid-fast bacteria in that disease independently. We both worked closely with micro-biologists, pathologists and microscopists. We both loved to play the piano, and to paint, and to read. We both wrote books and medical papers. We both were obsessed with the germ of cancer and devoted our lives to its study. Both of us challenged the medical and cancer establishments—Virginia with her vaccines and me with my accusations that AIDS is a man-made disease. She was my mentor, and I was her greatest supporter. Her research supported mine; and my research supported hers. Virginia's energy, despite her passing, is still a source of great strength for me.

In *The Bible*, God tells us we came from dust—and to dust we shall return, which is not terribly encouraging for those not confident about an afterlife. But what if dust contained the elements and building blocks that could remake life over and over again for all eternity? Isn't Earth basically a big pile of dust? Couldn't this be "God's little secret" He wants us to unravel?

What is life if it is not pulsating with cosmic energy? If the tiniest of life forms can exist and persist in meteors millions or billions of years old, and if we are composed and descended from the tiniest forms of life, why can't we live forever?

All we might need is a speck of dust and a little "faith" to ignite that spark of life that would get us going again.

CHAPTER FOUR

Microphotography of the Cancer Microbe

Part of the proof that the cancer microbe is implicated in the cause of cancer and certain other diseases like scleroderma, is based on the finding of pleomorphic bacteria within the diseased tissue itself (*in vivo*). Unfortunately, the "routine" stain (the hematoxylin-eosin stain) that pathologists use to make their tissue diagnosis is not suitable for demonstrating the microbe.

Virginia Livingston was the first to discover that the microbe was intermittently "acid-fast," either in tissue or in culture, or both. In acid-fast stained tissue sections examined at the highest power with the oil-immersion lens (1,000 times), a variety of pleomorphic forms can be demonstrated. These forms range from the tiniest "granules" (barely visible to the naked eye) up to larger round forms resembling "cocci" and approximating the size of ordinary staphylococci. Sometimes these round forms appear even larger, resembling the size and shape of yeast-like and fungal-like round spores. The largest of these forms are well known to pathologists as "Russell bodies." At present, pathologists do not consider Russell bodies as microbial in nature. However, the size and shape and staining characteristics of Russell bodies are compatible with "large body" forms of cell-wall-deficient bacteria, as described by some microbiologists. Unlike modern day pathologists, William Russell (himself a noted pathologist) described these forms in the late nineteenth century, and regarded them as "the cancer parasite."

Rarely, acid-fast rods resembling typical rod-forms of tuberculosis-type bacteria can be observed, particularly in scleroderma. I have only observed typical acid-fast rods in a cancer tumor on one occasion, in a reported case of an immunoblastic sarcoma in a man with AIDS.

The cancer microbe can be seen within the cells (intracellular) and outside the cells (extra-cellular), scattered in the connective tissue between the cells. As noted by Livingston, the microbe has a great affinity for "connective tissue." This is seen most clearly in the connective tissue of scleroderma.

In the following photos, various forms of the cancer microbe are presented in a variety of different cancers (breast cancer, prostate cancer, Hodgkin's disease, AIDS-related Kaposi's sarcoma), and in scleroderma. All the forms are photographed at a magnification of 1,000 times, the highest magnification available in the ordinary light microscope. Pleomorphic bacteria cultured from cancer may resemble staphylococci, corynebacteria-like and cocco-bacillary microbes ("diphtheroids"), mycobacteria, and fungal-like organisms. Obviously the viral-like forms are too small to be observed with light microscopy.

Figure 1   **SCLERODERMA**; rod-shaped
              bacteria in skin.

Figure 2   **SCLERODERMA**; cocco-
              bacilli (round and rod forms)
              cultured from scleroderma.

Figure 3   **KAPOSI'S SARCOMA**;
              coccoid bacteria in skin.

Figure 4 **PROSTATE CANCER**;
intracellular coccoid forms.

Figure 5 **HODGKIN'S DISEASE**;
granules, coccoid forms and small
Russell bodies in a cancerous
lymph node.

Figure 6 **HODGKIN'S DISEASE**; giant
solitary Russell body in a
cancerous lymph node.

Figure 7 **BREAST CANCER**; intra- and
extra-cellular coccoid forms in the
breast tumor.

Figure 8 **BREAST CANCER**; cocci
cultured from skin metastasis of
the original breast cancer.

Figure 1. **SCLERODERMA**: Tissue section showing acid-fast (red-stained) rods in the dermis of the skin. Fite stain, magnification 1,000 X in oil.

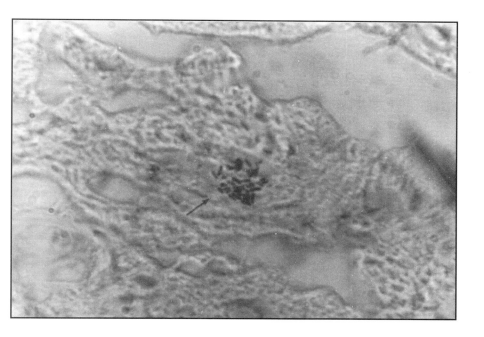

Figure 2. **SCLERODERMA**: Acid-fast stained smear from bacteriologic culture of skin showing cocco-bacillary non-acid-fast forms suggestive of "corynebacteria." Compare size and shape of these bacteria with the size and shape of the acid-fast bacteria observed *in vivo* in tissue in Fig. 1. Zeihl-Neelsen stain, magnification 1,000 X, in oil.

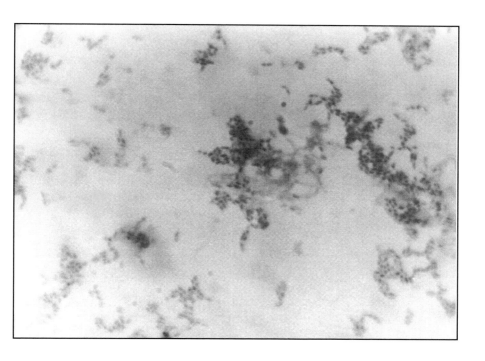

Figure 3. **KAPOSI'S SARCOMA** (AIDS-related): Arrows point to three foci of tiny intra-cellular and extra-cellular acid-fast granules and coccoid forms in the dermis of the skin. Fite (acid-fast) stain, magnification 1,000 X, in oil.

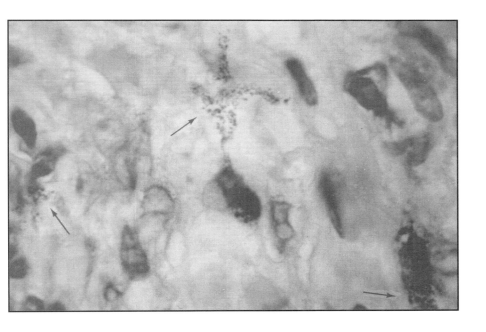

Figure 4. **PROSTATE CANCER**: Tissue section showing intra-cellular coccoid (round) forms in prostate cancer. Fite (acid-fast) stain, magnification 1,000 X, in oil.

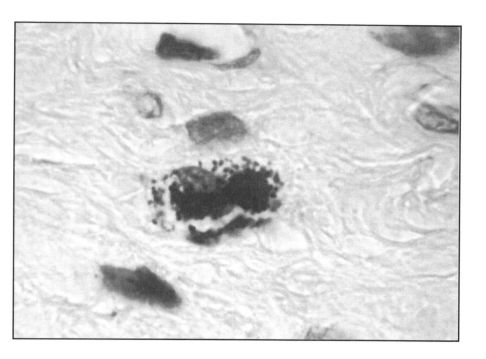

Figure 5. **HODGKIN'S DISEASE**: Tissue section of lymph node. Arrows point to two areas of tiny granules and larger round coccoid forms, consistent with "Russell bodies." These bodies were discovered in the late nineteenth century by pathologist Russell, who regarded them as "the parasite of cancer." These forms are also compatible with pleomorphic "cell-wall-deficient forms" of bacteria. The tissue is stained for bacteria with Gram's stain. Magnification 1000 X, in oil.

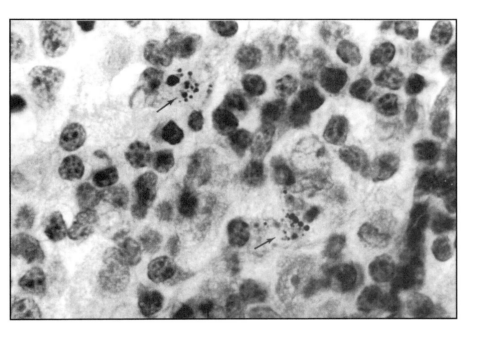

Figure 6. **HODGKIN'S DISEASE**: Same lymph node and stain (and magnification) showing giant Russell body in center. This very large structure is compatible with giant "L-forms," which are known forms of cell-wall-deficient bacteria. Such a large form is also in the size range of some fungal spores.

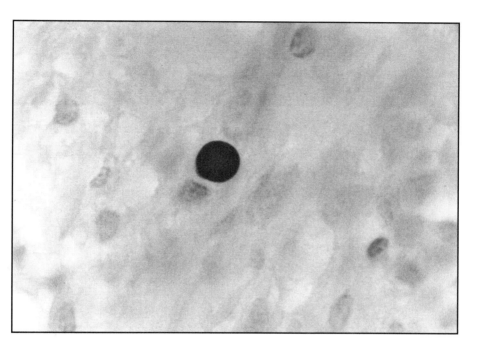

Figure 7. **BREAST CANCER**: Tissue section of breast cancer. Long arrows point to intra-cellular coccoid forms. Short arrows point to extra-cellular coccoid forms and minute granules. Intensified Kinyoun (acid-fast) stain, magnification 1,000 X, in oil.

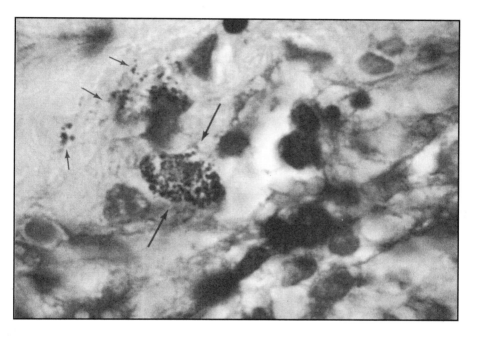

Figure 8. **BREAST CANCER**: Smear from bacteriolo-gical culture of skin showing metastatic breast cancer. The culture was identified as *Staphylococcus epidermidis*. Compare the size and shape of the cocci in culture to the coccoid forms seen in the original breast cancer and pictured in Fig. 7. Ziehl-Neelsen (acid-fast) stain, magnification 1,000 X, in oil.

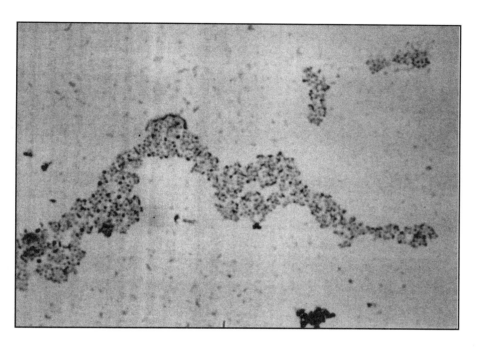

CHAPTER FIVE

The Cancer Microbe on the Internet

There is a wealth of information on the microbiology of cancer on the Internet.

The National Library of Medicine offers a website (http://www.ncbi.nlm.nih.gov/entrez/query.fcgi) called PubMed, which contains citations to scientific papers published in medical and scientific journals. These papers are also available for purchase. One can search for author's papers published as far back as the 1960s. For example, Virginia Livingston's papers from 1965 forward are cited, but there are no references to her early papers. To locate the titles of her papers, simply type in her last name and first initials in the search box. For Virginia Wuerthele-Caspe Livingston's papers, type in Livingston VW, and you will encounter six of her papers. Alexander-Jackson E has three citations. Seibert FB, 31; Diller IC, 22; and Cantwell AR, 30. You can also type in keywords in your search. For example, "Breast Cancer" gives 6,681 citations to various scientific journals.

An internet "search engine" such as www.google.com can also be very valuable when researching a particular topic or person. Simply enter the keywords in the search box. Typing in "cancer microbe" will direct you to 1,030 web pages; "cancer bacteria" (829); "Progenitor cryptocides" (380); "Virginia Livingston" (587).

You can "narrow" your search by using quotation marks around the person's name you are going to research. If you type in alan cantwell you will get 70,900 citations and encounter many "alans" and some "cantwells" that are not the author of this book. However, if you type in "alan cantwell" (with quotation marks) you will get 7,420 citations. Most will refer to my writings, but there are also several other "alan cantwells" in the world. To further refine your search, you can type in "alan cantwell" + "cancer microbe" (470 citations) or "alan cantwell" + cancer bacteria (570). On Google.com, "Progenitor cryptocides" will refer you to 381 websites.

Nanobac Labs has a website devoted to nanobacteria research. Nanobacteria have been found in heart and kidney disease, in various dermatologic diseases of unknown etiology, and have been detected in viral vaccines. (www.nanobaclabs.com/research/)

A number of papers by Alan Cantwell, M.D., featuring color microphotographs of cancer microbes in various diseases can be found at the website of the *Journal of Independent Medical Research* at www.joimr.org., hosted by editor Trevor Marshall.

There are many cancer microbe researchers of the past and present who have not been mentioned in this book, due to space requirements and restrictions. Among these researchers are the work of Raymond Royal Rife, Gaston Naessens, Guenther Enderlein, and Erik Enby, M.D. A www.google.com search of these people can provide additional information on various aspects of cancer microbe research.

INDEX of Proper Names

A NOTE ABOUT THE AUTHOR

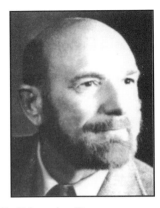

Alan Cantwell is a dermatologist and scientific researcher in the field of cancer and AIDS microbiology. He is a graduate of New York Medical College, and studied dermatology at the Long Beach Veteran's Administration Hospital in Long Beach, California. He was a member of the Dermatology Department at the Southern California Permanente Medical Group in Hollywood from 1965 until his retirement in 1994. He is the author of more than thirty published papers on cancer, AIDS, and other immunologic diseases, which have appeared in leading national and international peer-reviewed medical journals. His books include: *The Cancer Microbe*; *AIDS & the Doctors of Death*; *Queer Blood*; and *AIDS: The Mystery & the Solution*. He is a frequent contributor to *New Dawn* and *Paranoia* magazines, and lives in Hollywood, California, with his partner and five cats.

A NOTE ABOUT JOHN STEINBACHER

John Steinbacher is the Executive Director of the Cancer Federation and a former investigative reporter and TV/ radio commentator. He is the author of *Wayfarers of Fate*; *The Child Seducers*; and *An Inward Stillness and An Inward Healing*, among others. Mr. Steinbacher is a member of the 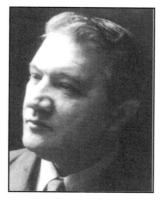 New York Academy of Sciences, the American Medical Writers Association, the American Society of Association Executives, and his biography appears in *Notable Americans*; and *Who's Who in America*. He has received honors from many noble institutions, including Rotary and the American Legion. In 1988 he was named an alumnus of the year by Pacific University for his philanthropic endeavors.

Also available from
ARIES RISING PRESS

THE CANCER MICROBE: The Hidden Killer in Cancer, AIDS, and Other Immune Diseases by Alan Cantwell covers a century of research into the infectious cause of cancer that has been suppressed and ignored by the medical establishment. Contains 19 photos (four in color) of the cancer microbe in breast cancer, lymphoma, AIDS-damaged tissue, lupus, scleroderma, etc. Softcover, 210 pp. $19.95

AIDS AND THE DOCTORS OF DEATH: An Inquiry into the Origin of the AIDS Epidemic by Alan Cantwell. A startling, fully-documented expose of AIDS as a man-made epidemic produced by a genetically engineered virus. Traces the origin of AIDS to vaccine experiments in which gays and African blacks unknowingly served as guinea pigs for genocidal purposes. Softcover, 239 pp. $14.95

QUEER BLOOD: The Secret AIDS Genocide Plot by Alan Cantwell. Further research showing why AIDS is a man-made disease and connecting its origin to biological warfare research. Winner of the Ben Franklin Book Award for Excellence. "A book and idea to be reckoned with."—*AIDS Book Review Journal.* Softcover, 168 pp. $12.95

AIDS: THE MYSTERY AND THE SOLUTION by Alan Cantwell. The most widely acclaimed classic bestseller showing the cancer microbe as the hidden co-factor necessary to produce full-blown AIDS. Includes chapters on sex and cancer, viruses and the immune system, AIDS in children, etc., and eight photos of the microbe in Kaposi's sarcoma and AIDS-damaged tissue. Softcover, 210 pp. $9.95

Order from your local bookseller or from Aries Rising Press, P.O. Box 29532, Los Angeles, CA 90029. Credit card orders available from Book Clearing House at 1-800-431-1579. Also available on-line at www.amazon.com. Email: alancantwell@sbc.global.net.